Adrenal Fatigue Diet & Action Plan

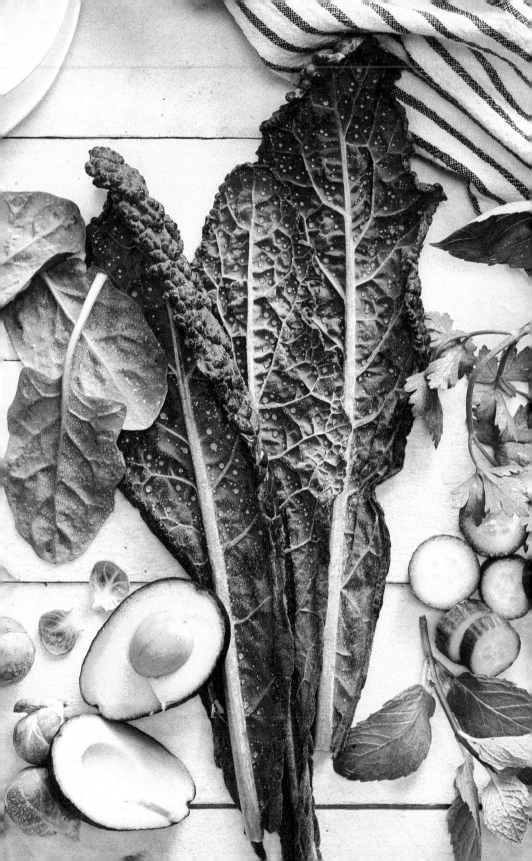

ADRENAL FATIGUE

diet & action plan

A 5-Week Meal Plan and
50+ Recipes to Fight Fatigue

Jennifer Maeng, MS, RD, CDN, CNSC

ROCKRIDGE
PRESS

Interior and Cover Designer: Rachel Haeseker
Art Producer: Sara Feinstein
Editors: Morgan Shanahan and Claire Yee

Photography © Andrew Purcell, cover; Thomas J. Story, p. ii, 18; Nadine Greeff/Stocksy, p. vi; Marija Vidal, p. xii–1; Laura Flippen, p. 30, 64–65; Cameron Whitman/Stocksy, p. 2, 126; Nadine Greeff, p. 66; Evi Abeler, p. 78; Hélène Dujardin, p. 88, 154; Darren Muir, p. 102; Alicia Cho, p. 114; Jennifer Chong, p. 134; Becky Stayner, p. 144.

Food styling by Carrie Purcell, cover

Author photo courtesy of © Rebecca Enis

ISBN: Print 978-1-64739-282-6 | eBook 978-1-64739-283-3

R0

I dedicate this book to my favorite sous chef, Connor, and my loudest cheerleader, Brian. And to all the patients who suffer from adrenal fatigue: I hope this book helps you take back your health in the most delicious possible way.

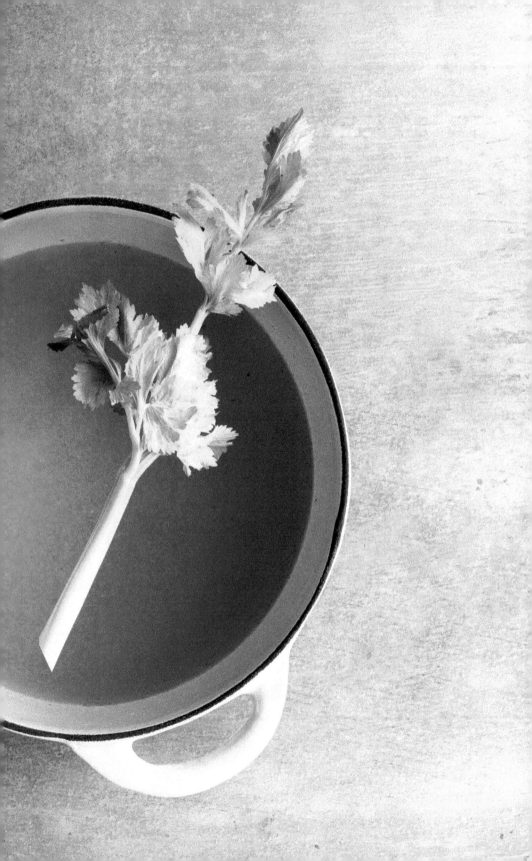

Contents

Introduction

My health and wellness private practice, Chelsea Nutrition, was named after the New York neighborhood I live in. It was important for me to open a practice that prioritized the communal, social, and personal relationships that we all have with food. I was formerly a clinical dietitian in a hospital. There, my role was usually responsive in nature, and most of the relationships I developed were professional. So when I first opened up private appointments for Chelsea Nutrition, I wasn't sure what types of clients I would meet—but I was excited to explore the individual connections that each person developed with what they ate.

Almost immediately, I noticed a pattern among clients—from their 20s to their 60s—coming in with similar symptoms related to various medical conditions, lifestyles, and eating habits. A large number of these clients had seen a primary doctor for their symptoms but were never given a clear diagnosis. Many were prescribed selective serotonin reuptake inhibitors (SSRIs) for anxiety or depression or were referred to an endocrinologist or gastroenterologist. Those referred to an endocrinologist were often prescribed thyroid hormones such as levothyroxine, and those referred to a gastroenterologist either left without treatment or had an endoscopy or colonoscopy, which usually didn't show clear, diagnosable signs of a medical condition. The host of other symptoms that they were experiencing weren't addressed. They weren't finding solutions, and they were frustrated.

Many clients complained of fatigue. Almost all were relying on caffeine to start the day, and many were relying on caffeine, sugary pick-me-ups, or both to get through the day, which led to poor gut health and weight gain. Weight gain, in most cases, spiraled them into low self-esteem and poor body image, creating a vicious cycle of emotional eating. They found themselves having entered a lifelong battle with weight.

Stress was another common symptom. Countless clients stated that they were constantly stressed and anxious about life, relationships, work, finances, kids, and health. They were not sleeping well, and they felt they had no time to take care of themselves. I remember speaking with a client who was clearly overburdened with family- and work-related anxiety and stress. When I gently asked her what she was doing for herself amid taking care of her family, she grew silent and then started crying. I have also seen many clients who suffered from stress-induced irritable bowel syndrome for years, causing crippling fear and anxiety around food and even about leaving the house. In some cases, weight loss was a huge problem—some reported 30 to 50 pounds of unintentional weight loss.

Psychological stress isn't the only cause of adrenal fatigue. There were also clients who didn't complain of high levels of stress but had an overall feeling of being unwell. From brain fog to chronic aches and pains, it was hard to pinpoint how I could help them until I learned more about their lifestyles and diets. What you eat and drink on a daily basis can cause physical stress responses in your body, and this can impact all of your bodily functions.

I wrote this book for those who feel frustrated about untreated adrenal fatigue symptoms to help you in the same way I help my clients. There is no one-size-fits-all solution to your health or to adrenal fatigue. Adrenal fatigue symptoms come in many forms, and eating for widely varying symptoms in addition to diet limitations may seem impossible. With this book, though, I can show you how to make realistic and sustainable changes so you feel your best in your own body.

Quick Start Guide

Finding proper treatments for adrenal fatigue and going from one doctor to another may feel like a long, frustrating journey. I wanted this cookbook to feel like just the opposite by telling you right up front what you should eat to feel good. The format of this book is different from a traditional cookbook in that it gives you a five-week meal plan (four weeks plus one bonus flare-up plan) to follow to help alleviate adrenal fatigue symptoms.

In chapters 1 and 2, I give you a quick rundown of what adrenal fatigue is and why you may be experiencing your current symptoms. Once you have a good idea about why adrenal fatigue is making you feel the way you feel and how food can help you, you may start to look at food as medicine or a toxin, rather than as pure calories.

In chapter 3, I will take you through your five-week meal plan, which includes detailed shopping lists, daily menus, and easy recipes with many substitution options. The primer week is about mentally preparing and seeing whether you can make a few small changes. From there, we slowly eliminate foods on the "avoid" list.

Chapters 4 through 11 are full of recipes that you can make independently or use as replacements in meal plans, which I encourage you to do if there are ever recipes you're not excited about. You should eat things you enjoy, even if the main goal is to address your medical condition.

Be realistic about the time you are able to or willing to invest in the kitchen. If you have a family, think about how to make this change a sustainable one for all of you. The key to success is to be realistic and honest with yourself. You want to set yourself up for success by planning a week that is manageable. Meal planning should not be another factor that adds stress to your life—if you're stressed, you'll aggravate your adrenal fatigue.

Carry snacks with you so you can avoid reverting to unhealthy choices. Review the Life Beyond the Meal Plan section (page 55) to learn how to make healthy food choices outside the meal plan, like during travel, dining out, and other events.

Last of all, don't give up! It may take you weeks or it may take you months, but with this book as your guide, you are building healthy eating habits for life. And remember that life happens, and there may be hurdles and slip-ups. Stay positive and get right back on the plan—that's how you'll see change happen.

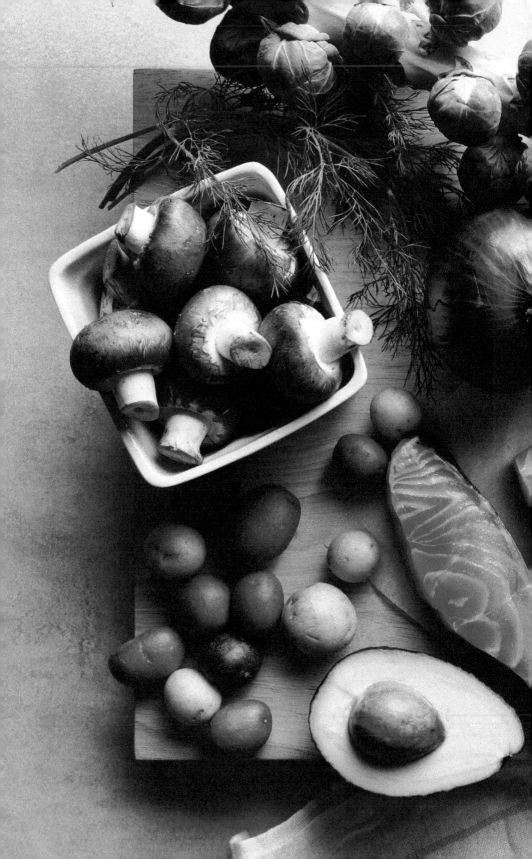

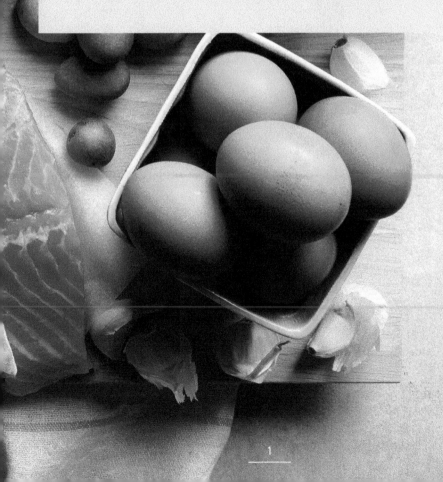

Part 1

Treating Adrenal Fatigue through Diet

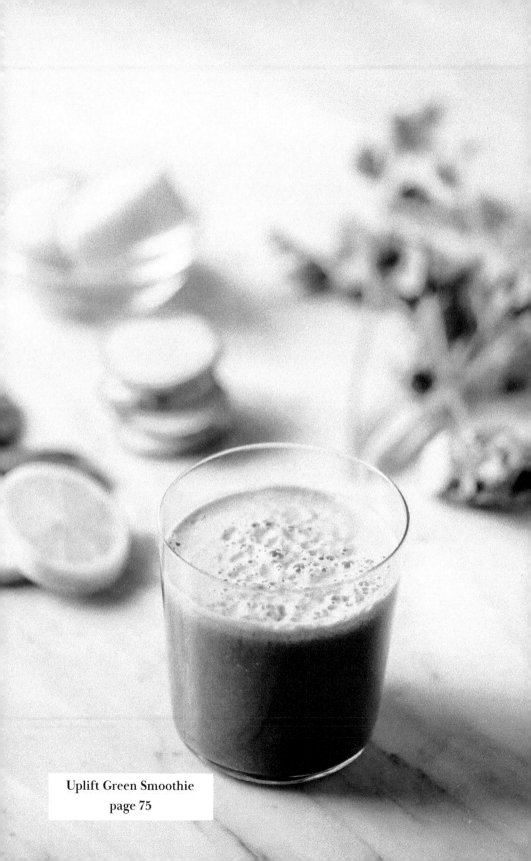

Uplift Green Smoothie
page 75

Chapter 1

What Is Adrenal Fatigue?

The definition of *healthy* is loaded, especially these days. It's a common misconception that being healthy equates to being thin. In reality, it's much more complicated than that. Your health is impacted by your social, emotional, physical, and mental well-being, and when any of these components is out of sync, optimal health can slip out of reach.

Among these components is adrenal fatigue. If not addressed, adrenal fatigue can lead to a host of chronic diseases that stem from physical, mental, and emotional exhaustion. This book will provide you with guidelines and resources to help you address adrenal fatigue and to teach you how to listen to and understand your body.

The adrenal system plays a large part in maintaining your body's metabolism, inflammatory responses, water and salt balance, blood sugar, energy levels, blood pressure, fertility, and many other essential functions. Your adrenal glands sit on top of your kidneys and are responsible for producing and regulating the release of stress response–related hormones. If your adrenal levels are too high—meaning excess hormones are being produced—you can be diagnosed with Cushing's disease. If the levels are too low, you can be diagnosed with Addison's disease. Both of these are extreme versions of adrenal dysfunction.

Many traditional doctors believe that your adrenal glands either work or don't—that there is no in-between. But that doesn't account for the broad range of adrenal dysfunction that can occur when your adrenals are compromised due to chronic stress on the body. This in-between condition is called adrenal fatigue.

Adrenal fatigue can lead to chronic exhaustion, body aches, an excessive need for caffeine, allergies, autoimmune disease, low libido, brain fog, weakness, salt and sweet cravings, increased appetite, weight gain and an inability to lose weight, and low immune function, among other problems that make you feel bad. Let's dive into the logistics of how this system works—or doesn't work—in your body.

So, You Feel Terrible

Adrenal fatigue is hugely impacted by levels of stress, as stress leads to inflammation in your body. Let's look at how your adrenal glands work when you're under stress. A stressful event can be anything from a life-threatening event to everyday stressors, such as work pressures or financial difficulties.

Imagine you're being chased by a lion. As you run for your life, your adrenal glands produce a hormone called adrenaline as the first response to the perceived threat. During this phase, your body will pause spending energy on nonurgent functions. Your reproduction or digestion will slow down, impacting not only your hormones but also your gut health. As the stress continues, adrenaline is no longer enough, and your body produces a stress hormone called cortisol.

Your body produces cortisol on a daily basis. Normally, it is at its highest level when you wake up in the morning and slowly decreases as you get ready for bed. The theory behind adrenal fatigue is that chronic low-level stress makes it impossible for the adrenal glands to release enough cortisol to keep up with the body's demand for it. It can become a vicious cycle—fatigue can cause stress, which can cause further fatigue.

It is so challenging to diagnose adrenal fatigue and find solutions to address it because adrenal fatigue is a newer chronic disease that still requires more research. Currently, there is no blood test that can measure smaller variations in adrenal function. Since medical doctors would make adrenal diagnoses based on the results of such a blood test, they cannot diagnose adrenal fatigue.

In addition, the symptoms of adrenal fatigue can vary greatly, from brain fog to food allergies to infertility. Many of my clients with adrenal fatigue have also been diagnosed with depression and prescribed medications for it, but this only addresses one of the side effects of adrenal fatigue. What about the sugar cravings, brain fog, food allergies, chronic exhaustion, aches, and pains?

The foods we eat help our bodies perform mentally and physically. Research has indicated that when we eat highly processed foods, our bodies may release messengers that cause inflammation, which can become chronic. By contrast, eating whole foods may help reduce inflammation in the body. Fruits and vegetables have antioxidants that may help our bodies recover from inflammation.

When Stress Makes You Sick and Causes More Stress

Chronic stress or inflammation in your body can directly impact your adrenal function. Stress management is vital to mitigating adrenal fatigue symptoms, avoiding flare-ups, and preventing comorbidities. Unfortunately, it's not always possible to remove the sources of stress from your life. It's helpful to identify your stressors so you can learn to recognize and control them. Here are a few things I like to suggest to my clients:

Breathing Exercises—When we are stressed and anxious, we tend to take rapid or shallow breaths, which can upset the balance of incoming oxygen and outgoing carbon dioxide. Relaxation breathing exercises can help us reset. One of my favorite techniques is called straw breathing (see the American Lung Association video in Resources on page 163). I recommend my clients do this daily and before they reach their peak stress level.   »

« **Meditation**—There are great apps that provide guided meditation, and many are free. My favorites are Meditation Studio, Calm, and Headspace. If you don't like one, try others until you find one that works for you.

Mood Booster—I like to ask my clients to make a list of things that can make them happy. Common ones I have heard are journaling, painting, cooking, running, and talking to friends. Keeping a list of these things can be a helpful reminder during stressful times.

The Main Symptoms of Adrenal Fatigue

Many of my clients with adrenal fatigue wake up feeling exhausted and continue to feel exhausted throughout the day. Here are some more detailed and additional examples of possible adrenal fatigue symptoms.

Exhaustion

When you're exhausted, you constantly feel weak, tired, or drained of ambition. Additional symptoms of exhaustion can include irritability, reduced immune function, and brain fog (see page 11). There is no strict set of diagnostic categories for exhaustion, so diagnosis can be challenging, but it's important to investigate any possible root causes. Many symptoms can be addressed in part with lifestyle changes and diet modification, which I will discuss further in chapter 2.

Depression

Depression affects how you feel and think and handle daily life. More common symptoms include persistent sadness, trouble sleeping or excessive sleeping, loss of energy, increased fatigue, weight gain or loss, difficulty concentrating or making decisions, and thoughts of self-harm or suicidal thoughts. In order for someone to be diagnosed with depression by a primary care provider (PCP) or a psychiatrist, depressive symptoms must persist for at least two weeks.

Blood tests may rule out other medical conditions that can contribute to depression. Depression is usually treated with psychotherapy, antidepressants, or a combination of the two. Antidepressants may cause side effects such as decreased alertness, nausea, headaches, high blood pressure, decreased libido, diabetes, and thoughts of suicide, so it's important to communicate with your doctor.

Sugar Cravings

There is no proper medical diagnosis for sugar or salt cravings other than binge eating disorder. However, adrenal hormones play an important role in regulating blood sugar levels. Without proper hormone function, your body cannot maintain a high enough blood sugar level, a condition called hypoglycemia. Hypoglycemia can cause sugar cravings—you need more energy fast, so you reach for pastries, candy, or other sugary, highly processed foods. Your body stores that energy for easy access when stress levels rise in the future—and this stored energy comes in the form of weight gain.

Poor Immune Function

Adrenal fatigue can lead to poor immune function due to an abnormal level of cortisol (high or low). If the body has too much or too little cortisol, the immune system cannot function properly because it no longer understands what to perceive as a threat. With poor immune function, you are more likely to get frequent colds, cold sores, infections, food sensitivities or allergies, digestive issues, and inflammation. Patients presenting with poor immune function are often prescribed antibiotics, steroids, or other medications to suppress symptoms and are sometimes left underdiagnosed for years.

Constant Need for Caffeine

People with adrenal fatigue often turn to stimulants for energy. Caffeine is one of the most utilized stimulant drugs in the world—it is found in coffee, tea, soda, energy drinks, chocolate, and over-the-counter pain medications. When you ingest caffeine, it sends a signal from your central nervous system telling the adrenal gland to produce adrenaline and cortisol. If you drink multiple cups of coffee per day, you can overwork your adrenal glands and put your body in constant fight-or-flight mode. Excessive caffeine consumption has been linked to worsened PMS and menopause symptoms, insomnia, gastrointestinal distress, and acid reflux disease.

Mental Health Check-In:
When It's More than a Symptom

Anyone can become depressed, and there are both mental and physical symptoms of depression, including but not limited to feeling worthless or hopeless, loss of enjoyment of everyday activities, aches and pains, digestive issues, insomnia, or excessive sleeping. If you believe you may be depressed, it is important to get proper assessment by a medical professional, such as your PCP or a psychiatrist.

Depression caused by adrenal fatigue and depression caused by genetic, environmental, psychological, or other biological factors may present similar symptoms, but treatment will not always be the same. As a dietitian, I first thoroughly interview my clients to understand the root cause of their depression before I make recommendations.

As an example, my clients with adrenal fatigue–induced irritable bowel syndrome (IBS) often complain of frustration, anxiety, brain fog, and depression (read more about IBS on page 11). When interviewing them, I ask: Is your depression presenting as a symptom of IBS, or did it exist prior to the onset of IBS? Their answer will determine their treatment route.

In the case of IBS, there can be a lot of anxiety around choosing the right foods, unexpected bowel movements, difficulty focusing at work, intimacy, and social life. These stressors can lead to depression—but the root cause is IBS. When depression presents this way, I can guide my clients in making modifications to their diet and lifestyle habits to reduce IBS symptoms and thereby relieve the triggers for depression. Of course, this approach must be combined with proper mental health treatment.

An important note: Those who have adrenal fatigue symptoms in addition to a psychological condition (such as an eating disorder, trauma, or suicidal ideation) should not try to resolve their condition with the adrenal fatigue diet. In these cases, it is crucial to seek psychiatric therapy and proper medical treatment.

Managing Symptoms

As a dietitian, I help people manage their symptoms with food. This often involves working closely with other medical professionals to help my clients from multiple angles. I want to emphasize that not all symptoms can be fully addressed with food, but food can help set you on the right path. Here are a few dietary and cognitive tips you should follow if you are experiencing adrenal fatigue:

Remove caffeine from your diet—I know this is a tough one to give up for many, but given its direct impact on your adrenal glands, I recommend that you stay away. One trick that has worked very well for my clients is tracking their water intake. I rarely meet a new client who is meeting their hydration needs. The recommended daily fluid intake published by the National Academies of Sciences, Engineering, and Medicine is about 11 cups (2.7 liters) for women and about 16 cups (3.7 liters) for men (including fluids in all foods and beverages)—unless you have a medical condition that requires fluid restriction. Once my clients focus on meeting their fluid intake, they realize how much less coffee they need to drink.

Find relaxation—When my clients say they are exhausted, I ask them to walk me through their typical day. Often, their days are filled with back-to-back meetings and their nights are filled with business dinners, social events, or long hours sitting in front of the TV. This all-too-typical lifestyle can take a toll on your health, regardless of your age. Your body needs time to relax in order to repair. Relaxation can come in many forms, such as getting to bed even a little earlier, reducing screen time and exposure to blue light, and meditating.

Be mindful of your gut and brain—Your gut is closely connected to your brain. Gut health can impact your mood, concentration, brain fog, and immune function—your gut contains about 70 percent of the cells that make up your immune system. There is growing evidence that when you consume foods that irritate your gut, your gut sends signals to your central nervous system that can trigger changes in your mood and brain function. We will discuss foods that support (and don't support) gut health in chapter 2.

Comorbid Diagnosis: Complicating Complications

Many people who experience adrenal fatigue experience **comorbidity**—the presence of two or more conditions at the same time. Having adrenal fatigue with comorbidity makes it difficult to properly diagnose and cope with adrenal fatigue. Some comorbidities require medical attention, and medications prescribed for the comorbid condition may exacerbate adrenal fatigue symptoms. Here are a few examples of commonly seen comorbidities and the dietary challenges they may present.

Low Blood Pressure

Different organs and hormones regulate our blood pressure, and the adrenal glands are one of them. When the adrenal glands produce insufficient levels of cortisol, it can lead to low blood pressure (hypotension). Symptoms of low blood pressure include dizziness, lightheadedness, nausea, dehydration, unusual thirst, lack of concentration, and fatigue. Doctors usually monitor blood pressure through routine visits and sometimes prescribe medication. Dietary modifications, like monitoring hydration and nutrient intake, can help regulate low blood pressure, but treatment should be highly individualized on a case-by-case basis.

Hypoglycemia

When your stress level is high and your adrenaline and cortisol are elevated, your body will require immediately accessible energy to keep up with increased demand. In the later stages of adrenal fatigue, your cortisol level starts to drop off and can no longer help regulate blood sugar levels. In turn, blood sugar levels can crash.

When your blood sugar drops, causing hypoglycemia, your body craves the simple carbohydrates found in bread, cookies, chips, and candy. These foods will raise your blood sugar quickly, but they have poor nutritional content, and the energy won't last. Worse, they can also exacerbate IBS, brain fog, Hashimoto's, and even fibromyalgia. Incorporating more fiber—particularly soluble fiber—into your diet will slow the absorption of sugar and improve blood sugar control.

Insomnia

Stress levels and sleep quality are interconnected. Stress levels affect the hypothalamic-pituitary-adrenal axis (HPA axis), which is responsible for regulating the sleep-wake cycle through the secretion of hormones like melatonin. Disrupted sleep and insomnia can cause the HPA axis to malfunction, creating an endless cycle of stress-induced metabolic abnormalities. Metabolic disturbances can in turn lead to fatigue and sleepiness during the day, which can lead to caffeine dependence, which can feed back into the cycle of insomnia.

Managing stress can support improving sleep quality, as can exercise, meditation, and diet. Foods high in tryptophan, such as fish, eggs, nuts, seeds, and complex carbohydrates, such as quinoa or brown rice, can boost the neurotransmitter serotonin, which is responsible for the regulation of sleep, appetite, pain inhibition, and mood.

Brain Fog

"Brain fog" refers to periods of forgetfulness and impaired cognition related to an inability to process information. Patients with brain fog have difficulty taking in information, focusing, and remembering things. Brain fog can stem from functional or structural damage to the brain due to chronic fatigue, exhaustion, and nutritional deficiency.

Unfortunately, brain fog is hard to diagnose and therefore hard to treat. In addition to sleep and stress management, brain fog can be addressed by giving your body the nutrients it needs to function. These include water, complex carbohydrates, fruits, nuts, seeds, and fatty fish, such as salmon.

Irritable Bowel Syndrome (IBS) and Other Gastrointestinal (GI) Disorders

When cortisol levels are imbalanced—as they are in adrenal fatigue—digestion and absorption become compromised. This is because cortisol activates the sympathetic nervous system, which controls the body's fight-or-flight response. When cortisol activates the sympathetic nervous system, it deactivates the parasympathetic nervous system, which controls the body's unconscious actions, including digestion and absorption. When the parasympathetic nervous system is deactivated, digestion cannot occur—so indigestion occurs. This can cause the gastrointestinal tract to become irritated and inflamed, as in IBS patients.

When the GI tract is chronically inflamed, as it is during adrenal fatigue, it cannot fully function. This may lead to other conditions, such as IBS, Hashimoto's, fibromyalgia, toxin overload, and depression. Good dietary habits can improve GI tract function, immune system function, and even mental health, including depression.

Stress management and dietary patterns are critical in the treatment and management of symptoms of IBS. Certain foods such as gluten, sugar substitutes, dairy, carbonated beverages (sodas or flavored sparkling drinks), caffeine, alcohol, fried foods, and cruciferous vegetables can further irritate the GI tract and exacerbate symptoms of IBS and fibromyalgia. On the bright side, clients who follow a strict diet (referred to as low-FODMAP) under the guidance of an experienced registered clinical dietitian can learn to control and alleviate symptoms and flare-ups.

Food Sensitivities

In adrenal fatigue, abnormal cortisol levels can result in an overactive immune system and an increased inflammatory response. In an overactive immune system, your body can't tell the difference between normal body health and real threats to the body.

Food allergies occur when the immune system perceives an ingested food as harmful to the body, even if it isn't. Food sensitivities occur when the body has difficulty digesting certain foods. Both result in inflammation as the immune system tries to protect the body. Avoiding food triggers and following a diet plan to prevent and reduce inflammation can help prevent flare-ups.

Hashimoto's Disease

Hashimoto's disease is an autoimmune disorder in which the thyroid gland becomes inflamed, causing hypothyroidism, which is when the thyroid gland produces insufficient hormones to help the body function. Hypo-thyroidism can cause a domino effect, resulting in various issues, including cardiovascular disease, impaired glucose control, and hyperglycemia (high blood sugar).

Hashimoto's disease is treated with prescribed thyroid hormone replacement therapy, but diet can also play a significant role in preventing and reducing chronic inflammation. A diet high in antioxidants (found in fruits, vegetables, nuts, and seeds) may help reduce inflammation and slow the progression of the disease.

Fibromyalgia and Chronic Pain

Fibromyalgia is a chronic condition identified by the primary symptoms of widespread pain, tenderness, and fatigue. Other symptoms include trouble sleeping, impaired cognition, brain fog, and chronic fatigue. Fibromyalgia is notoriously difficult to diagnose and treat because fatigue can be a side effect of numerous health conditions.

Currently, there is no diagnostic test for fibromyalgia, and diagnosis is done through examining patient symptoms and ruling out other conditions. Moreover, patients with fibromyalgia may have one or more existing comorbidities, such as IBS or chronic fatigue syndrome. A well-balanced diet of protein, carbohydrates, and fat is most important for managing fatigue.

Toxin Overload

Toxins in the body can come from a number of sources, including chemicals in polluted air, heavy metals (like mercury and lead), cleaning solutions, paints, antibiotics, and even the foods we eat. When ingested, toxins can be stored in our blood, fat tissues, organs, and bones, sometimes leading to metabolic dysfunction.

Studies (including one published in the *British Medical Journal*) have indicated that prolonged exposure to toxins can not only lower thyroid hormone levels, metabolic rate, and fat-burning abilities but also alter hormonal and neuroregulatory mechanisms in the body. Symptoms of toxin overload include hormonal imbalance, unusual appetite, inflammation, weight gain or trouble with weight loss, chronic fatigue, sensitivities to chemicals and food, skin infections, and gastrointestinal issues.

Although no single diet can help repair damage done by prolonged exposure to toxins, foods that help regulate and maintain a healthy gut can help combat symptoms of toxin overload. Following dietary guidelines will also help address Hashimoto's disease, IBS, depression, and chronic pain.

I Got 99 Health Problems: FAQ

It's important to start your journey to address adrenal fatigue with a medical professional who can ensure you are addressing medical symptoms, such as depression, Hashimoto's, and IBS, in the right order. Here are some frequently asked questions when it comes to these comorbidities:

Q: *How do medications complicate things?*
A: Depending on the severity of IBS symptoms, antibiotics or steroid treatment will be required to reduce inflammation. Antibiotics often wipe out all your good *and* bad gut bacteria, which can alter your gut health unless managed properly. This can lead to depression, food sensitivities, brain fog, and even chronic pain. If managed properly, though, you can see change in just two to four weeks.

Q: *What happens if I am misdiagnosed?*
A: Misdiagnosis is common. I have had many clients who were diagnosed with Lyme disease, which can present with similar symptoms. In the event of a misdiagnosis, medications such as antidepressants, steroids, antibiotics, and thyroid hormone therapies may have been prescribed to address symptoms without considering the root cause. Medications can have side effects, which may in turn affect your gut.

Q: *Can supplements help?*
A: Supplements are not considered drugs, so they are not regulated according to FDA standards. Because of the lack of regulation, it is difficult to assess how medications may interact with supplements—for this reason, I hesitate to recommend them. Before taking any supplements, work with medical professionals to ensure there is sufficient evidence to support their supposed benefits.

Q: *Can people with adrenal fatigue feel their best again?*
A: Yes! The purpose of this book is to help you feel your best again by making diet and lifestyle changes specific to your adrenal fatigue symptoms and comorbidities. It won't happen overnight, but with persistence and dedication, I believe you can feel better.

Personalize Your Approach

The symptoms of adrenal fatigue vary widely. This book is put together with a large number of symptoms in mind. It includes easy-to-follow plans that allow you to make adjustments to fit your specific symptoms and comorbidities.

I believe that treatment through diet should be flexible and customizable. I try to spend as much time as possible understanding my clients' lifestyles, health concerns, and health goals to make sure my recommendations and plans are individualized. Throughout the recipes, I provide numerous shortcuts, substitution options, and other modifications. Use the Recipe Index by Symptom (page 164) and the Ingredient Index (page 169) to choose recipes that work best for your body's needs—remember, you are your own best advocate!

Each recipe is labeled with adrenal fatigue comorbidities and symptoms so that you can easily pinpoint recipes that will work for you. All the recipes are created with adrenal fatigue in mind. Chapter 2 includes more information about the recipe labels (page 28).

Optimize Your Care Providers

Multiple health care professionals can take part in diagnosing and treating adrenal fatigue. Each professional plays a specific role in helping you understand your symptoms and comorbidities.

PCP

Your PCP may want to test your cholesterol level, red blood cell count (to rule out anemia), and thyroid-stimulating hormone (TSH) and thyroid (to measure thyroid function). Other testing may include an insulin-induced hypoglycemia test (to see how the HPA axis responds to stress), an ACTH stimulation test (to measure the stress response of the adrenal glands), or a urine test (to measure hormone profiles and cortisol patterns).

If your PCP conducts these tests and finds any abnormalities, they can also refer you to specialists (rheumatologists, endocrinologists, psychiatrists, and registered dietitians) to limit stress triggers and adrenal fatigue exacerbation. In patients with adrenal fatigue, though, the results from these tests may show that symptoms do not appear critical.

Rheumatologist

Rheumatologists specialize in diagnosing and treating musculoskeletal disease and autoimmune disease that can impact the muscles, joints, and bones. Rheumatologists can diagnose and treat adrenal fatigue comorbidities such as rheumatoid arthritis, chronic pain, and fibromyalgia.

Overproduction of cortisol and androgen can lead to poor bone growth and development and elevated risk of bone fracture and bone loss. Those with rheumatic disease are also at a higher risk for fibromyalgia and chronic pain.

Endocrinologist

Endocrinologists are specialists who treat diseases and conditions related to the endocrine system, which handles the secretion and regulation of hormones. If hormone tests ordered by your PCP come back with abnormal results, you may be referred to an endocrinologist to further assess your adrenal function and possible underlying adrenal disease. In the case of adrenal insufficiency, endocrinologists can help regulate hormone levels through treatments such as hormone replacement therapy.

Mental Health Specialist

Stress management is integral to healthy adrenal function. Chronic stressors, such as financial strain, job insecurity, parenting issues, and even relationship problems, are often ignored and considered a part of life one should just accept. But even seemingly typical daily stressors may be linked to problems with adrenal gland function. A licensed psychiatrist or psychologist can help identify stress triggers and find ways to manage your stressors.

Dietitian

Registered dietitians (RDs) are trained professionals who can help assess and analyze your diet and lifestyle to guide you through managing adrenal fatigue. They can prescribe dietary modifications to help manage or even decrease symptoms and address digestive issues.

For patients with adrenal fatigue who also experience disordered eating, RDs can incorporate mindful eating therapy to build healthier relationships with food. For those with high cortisol levels, RDs can provide support with an anti-inflammatory diet to help reduce inflammation that may aggravate adrenal function. RDs can also address and treat nutrition- and lifestyle-related comorbidities that may occur—that's where I come in. I hope that this book gives you a helpful introduction to the work a hired dietitian might do.

I understand that not everyone has the resources to address their adrenal fatigue on their own, so I have put together thorough, step-by-step guidelines on how to begin tackling it.

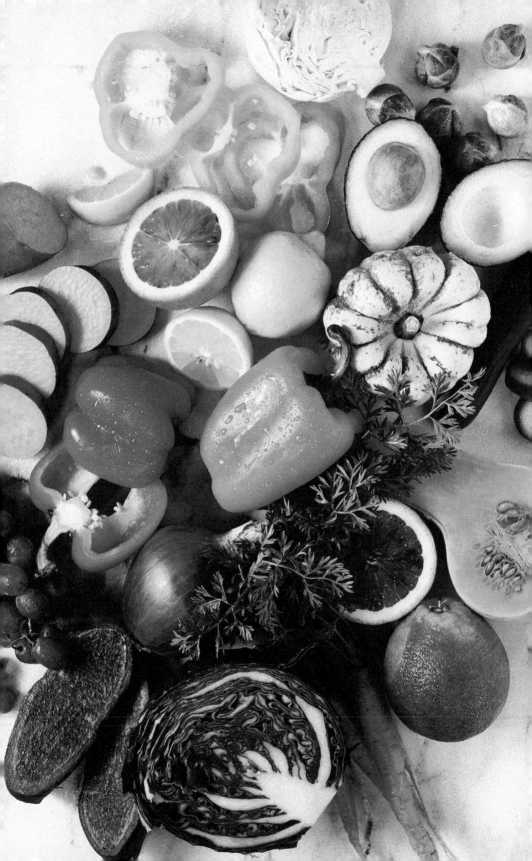

Chapter 2

How Your Diet Can Impact Your Symptoms

Nutrition is complicated and interconnected with every aspect of the body. When it comes to diet and health, many people rely heavily on internet search engines to find answers. There is so much conflicting information about adrenal fatigue and the adrenal diet in books and on television, blogs, and social media. My goal is to help you understand the relationship between food and bodily function to eliminate confusion and fear around eating.

Start Where You Are

Changing your diet and eating habits isn't easy. Your eating patterns, food preferences, and relationship with food have been shaped over many years, and overnight change is unrealistic. Many of my new clients want to make extreme changes from day one, and I always encourage them to start slowly and add on as they succeed. This incremental change will help make the diet change more permanent and sustainable.

Let's be honest here—stress surrounding food is common. Constant worry about which foods you "shouldn't" eat and guilt about making the "wrong" choices can keep stress levels high—and stress comes with its own list of health issues. When pursuing health, stress is the opposite of what we need.

Here's what I suggest: Think about why you want to try the adrenal fatigue diet. (Many of my clients say they want to feel like themselves again.) Instead of focusing on food that is not allowed, think about the foods that will help you feel better. I'll start you out with a basic plan to set you up for success.

Food: It Impacts Everything

When you start out on the adrenal fatigue diet in this book, I will help you ease into making incremental changes. We'll remove one-third of the foods to avoid each week. You won't start a full-fledged adrenal fatigue diet until Week 3 of the meal plan. There are a few specific foods that are associated with poor adrenal function.

Foods to Avoid

Here is a list of the foods you should avoid due to their connection to adrenal fatigue.

Processed foods—Inflammation triggers include sugar, salt, and highly processed fats (canola, rapeseeds, hydrogenated oils); refined grains; chemical flavorings; and preservatives.

Refined or artificial sugar—Your body is not able to break down and use artificial sweeteners or refined sugar as caloric sources. In addition to causing weight gain, natural, refined, or artificial sweeteners have been shown to cause inflammation by altering gut microbiota, according to research published in *The American Journal of Clinical Nutrition*.

Gluten—Found in wheat products, gluten can cause gut inflammation and autoimmune response. If you consume gluten and have thyroid issues, a protein found in gluten (called gliadin) can cause the body to attack the thyroid gland.

Dairy—Dairy is a common trigger for gastrointestinal distress, possibly due to environmental toxins, hormones, enzyme deficiencies, or antibiotics. Research on the environmental issues related to dairy has been published by the Food and Agriculture Organization of the United Nations.

Soy—Although soy is packed with protein, fiber, vitamins, and minerals, its estrogen-like compounds (isoflavone and phytoestrogen) may affect thyroid hormone function. Soy may act as an endocrine disruptor in the body, mimicking estrogen and causing hormone imbalance.

Red meats—Red meat has been shown to increase inflammatory markers such as C-reactive protein, according to a study published by the *European Journal of Nutrition*.

Alcohol and caffeine—Alcohol registers in the body as a toxin. Both alcohol and caffeine are stimulants that have a direct impact on the HPA axis.

Trigger foods (individualized)—Avoid foods that you know trigger symptoms of adrenal fatigue for you personally.

Healing Foods

Here is a list of common adrenal fatigue symptoms and healing foods that combat each one:

Combat caffeine overload with water—Coffee is high in antioxidants and can boost metabolic rate, but caffeine can also exacerbate adrenal fatigue. I recommend working toward meeting your hydration needs with water for more energy.

Combat exhaustion with vitamins B and C—B vitamins help turn food into energy for the body, and vitamin C aids in tissue repair. Foods high in vitamin B include salmon, avocado, broccoli, lentils, and eggs. Foods high in vitamin C include citrus fruits, strawberries, and cantaloupes.

Combat brain fog with magnesium and omega-3 fatty acids—Magnesium can improve circadian rhythm and help regulate neurotransmitters. It is found in green vegetables and nuts. Omega-3s are crucial for normal brain function and mood and are found in fatty fish, walnuts, and chia seeds.

Combat poor immune function with probiotics and vitamin E— Vitamin E is an antioxidant that can help prevent damage to cells, and probiotics may help boost immune cells and aid in gut health. Vitamin E is found in leafy green vegetables, almonds, and sunflower seeds, and probiotics are found in yogurt, kimchi, and sauerkraut.

Combat depression with vitamin D—Studies, including one published in *The British Journal of Psychiatry*, show an association between low vitamin D levels and depression. Foods high in vitamin D include salmon, tuna, and fortified plant-based milk.

Feeling Better through Food

The food we eat affects how we feel mentally and physically. Addressing adrenal fatigue symptoms through diet will help reduce inflammation and provide your body with the proper nourishment it needs. Let me walk you through a couple of alternative scenarios to help you get through the day:

Morning routine—In the morning, you're exhausted, even though you just slept for six to eight hours. You go to the kitchen to make a cup of coffee or two. You have no energy to make breakfast, so you get ready for work and rush out of the house. On the way to work, you grab a pastry or a bagel and eat at your desk as you check your email (or you skip breakfast altogether).

Here's what I suggest instead: First thing in the morning, drink a large glass of room-temperature water with a squeeze of fresh lemon juice or a tablespoon of apple cider vinegar. Prepare a bag of berries and two hard-boiled eggs the night before so you can grab them for breakfast. Drink another glass of plain water before you leave the house. If you don't have time to eat at home, take your breakfast to go—eat at your desk before you start checking your email.

Lunch—For lunch, rather than choosing high-carbohydrate foods like a burrito or pasta (and going through a subsequent blood sugar crash), choose high-fiber meals that contain protein and plant-based fat, such as a salad or brown rice bowl with lean protein and plenty of non-starchy vegetables.

This combination will help you stay full longer and will prevent your blood sugar from crashing midafternoon.

Midafternoon cravings—You might be tempted to have another cup of coffee and a bag of chips. Instead of coffee, I suggest a large glass of water or another naturally decaffeinated beverage. Instead of chips, I recommend a snack with protein, fiber, and fat, such as an apple with almond or cashew butter, or a handful of seed crackers with hummus.

Try your best not to fixate on choosing foods that other people think are healthy—you know your body best. Focus on staying connected to your own symptoms and seeking out foods that you know will help you.

A Healing Kitchen

I spend a lot of time convincing my clients to stop labeling foods as "good" or "bad." When you criticize yourself for eating "bad" food, the so-called bad food can become a point of fixation. I urge you to instead think about foods in terms of how they can make you feel. This will help make your kitchen into a healing space to prepare food that makes you feel good and satisfies your cravings.

Pantry

High-quality ingredients make a dish shine. Just because something is labeled as "natural" or "healthy" doesn't mean it is. Always read the Nutrition Facts panel, look for items with short ingredient lists and few processed ingredients, and choose organic when possible. When purchasing canned foods, such as tomatoes and beans, always look for "no salt added" and "BPA-free lining." If a can is dented, throw it away to avoid harmful bacteria (such as *Clostridium botulinum*, which can lead to a rare but serious illness, botulism). These are items I recommend you always have in your pantry:

Oils—coconut oil, extra-virgin olive oil, sesame oil

Vinegars—apple cider vinegar, balsamic vinegar, Champagne vinegar, sherry vinegar

Sauces and spreads—coconut aminos, Dijon mustard, nut and seed butters (cashew, almond, peanut, or sunflower), tahini

Canned or boxed goods (always unsalted, BPA-free)—beans (chickpeas, black beans, kidney beans), coconut milk, chicken broth, pumpkin, tomatoes, tomato paste

Dry goods—brown rice, buckwheat flour, chia seeds, chickpea flour, coconut flour, dried seaweed, flaxseed, gluten-free oats and oat flour, gluten-free pasta (brown rice, lentil, or chickpea), lentils, quinoa, unsweetened cocoa powder; be sure to always check ingredient packaging to ensure foods were processed in a completely gluten-free facility

Spices—bay leaves, black pepper (preferably whole peppercorns in a grinder), cinnamon, cloves, coriander, ground cumin, cumin seed, kosher salt, red pepper flakes, alcohol-free pure vanilla extract

Other—aluminum-free baking powder, baking soda

Refrigerator

I recommend shopping for produce once or twice a week to ensure freshness. You can prepare your meals in parts—for example, if you have three or four servings of grains and vegetables cooked in advance, you will always have 50 to 100 percent of your meals ready to use in a simple grain bowl or a warm salad, soup, or side. Sauces and dressings can also be prepared ahead of time and refrigerated, sometimes for up to a few weeks.

Vegetables (excluding alliums)—artichokes, asparagus, beets, bell peppers, broccoli, Brussels sprouts, cabbage, carrots, cauliflower, celery, cucumber, eggplant, fennel, green beans, jicama, kale, mushrooms, parsnips, radishes, spinach, winter squash (like butternut and kabocha), sweet potatoes, tomatoes, watercress, zucchini

Alliums—garlic, leeks, scallions, shallots, yellow onions (if you have IBS, avoid onions, garlic, and shallots, and only use the green parts of leeks and scallions)

Fruits—apples, bananas, blackberries, blueberries, gooseberries, kiwis, lemons, limes, melons, oranges, peaches, plums, raspberries, strawberries, tangerines

Fresh herbs—parsley, cilantro, fresh ginger, mint, basil

Plant-based protein—eggs (cage-free, pasture-raised preferred), plant-based yogurt (such as almond or coconut), unsweetened plant-based milk (oat or almond recommended)

Freezer

Frozen fruits and vegetables are absolutely okay to buy! They're more affordable, and they're picked and packaged at peak season, so they retain more nutrients. If your schedule and plans won't allow you to shop for produce every week, it makes more sense to buy frozen vegetables to have on hand.

Fruits—blueberries, pineapple, raspberries, strawberries

Vegetables—asparagus, cauliflower, bell peppers, broccoli, butternut squash, spinach

Nuts and seeds (unsalted)—almonds, cashews, pecans, pine nuts, pumpkin seeds (pepitas), sunflower seeds, sesame seeds, walnuts (Tip: Store nuts in your freezer to keep them fresh—they are high in fat content and can go rancid in the pantry.)

Animal-source protein—Choose lean proteins, like chicken, turkey, or seafood. Keeping protein in the freezer will save you the trouble of shopping multiple times a week. Move it to the refrigerator before you leave the house in the morning, and it will be thawed by the time you get home.

> **Seafood**—cod, rainbow trout, salmon, shrimp, sole

> **Poultry (organic and free-range)**—boneless, skinless chicken breasts and thighs; ground turkey

Cooking Equipment

You don't need a lot of cooking tools to get started. For me, a mini food processor and pressure cooker are essential and save me a lot of time in the kitchen. I've created a list of essential and nonessential cooking appliances. Don't worry if you don't have all of the tools listed—the recipes in this book can be made with basic kitchen tools and equipment.

Essentials

The following items are essentials to prepare the recipes in this book and are a great start to a well-equipped kitchen.

Appliances—miniature or standard-size food processor, high-speed blender, pressure cooker or electric multicooker such as the Instant Pot

Pots and pans—small saucepan with a lid (1-quart), medium saucepan with a lid (4-quart), large Dutch oven (6- to 8-quart), nonstick skillet with a lid (10- to 12-inch), small skillet with a lid (8-inch), two to four large (18-inch) rimmed baking sheets (or the largest size that will fit in your oven)

Utensils—kitchen scissors, chef's knife, paring knife, serrated knife, heat-resistant flat silicone spatula, wooden mixing spoon, ladle, tongs, fine-mesh sieve or strainer

Miscellaneous—grater, Microplane, colander, measuring spoons and cups, mixing bowls (small, medium, large)

Nice-to-Haves

These items are nice to have, but most recipes in this book can be prepared without them.

* Cast-iron skillet
* Handheld frother
* Rice cooker
* Spiralizer
* Waffle iron

About the Meal Plans

Making changes to your eating habits overnight isn't easy, and overnight change isn't sustainable, either. This plan is not a fad diet to try for a few weeks or a month. It can take between six months and a year to reset and heal your adrenal glands. In order to begin seeing changes with a diet, I generally recommend my clients follow a strict plan for four to six weeks.

For my clients with adrenal fatigue, I recommend an even longer plan. This is a commitment to yourself and to your body, but if you stick with it, it will end in good results.

As discussed earlier, adrenal fatigue comes with many different symptoms and comorbidities, and not everyone's experience is the same. The meal plans are designed not only to help alleviate adrenal fatigue but also to be customizable to your unique set of symptoms and dietary restrictions.

I will also ease you into making changes so you don't feel deprived of your favorite foods. For example, maple syrup is still incorporated in the first week's meal plan so you can wean yourself off sugar. If you don't eat sugar as it is, feel free to go without it from the beginning.

This meal plan is designed to make it easier for you to make positive changes toward health, not to add stress or make you feel deprived. Before you begin, think about how you can continue to motivate yourself to make long-lasting changes and continue on the path to success.

About the Recipes

The recipes in this book have been tested to ensure they are easy to follow, packed with flavor, and meet the needs of various adrenal fatigue symptoms, food sensitivities, and food preferences. The ingredients used are easy to find and repeat often throughout the book. The recipes are also easy to modify and personalize to fit individual needs.

Types of Dishes

All the recipes in this book use fresh, simple, and accessible ingredients to maximize nutrients and make cooking exciting and fun. Even if you're new to cooking, these recipes will start to get easier after just a week or two. Most recipes make multiple servings (usually between 2 and 6) so that you'll have leftovers to eat the next day. Many of these recipes have been tested and approved by my amazing clients, and I hope you enjoy them as much as they have.

Recipes by Symptom

Each recipe is labeled with the specific symptoms it can help address. This book also provides a Recipe Index by Symptom (page 164) so you can look up your symptoms and easily find recipes. Here is a list of the recipe labels used:

Brain Fog—In addition to facilitating better sleep, these recipes will help reduce brain fog and support brain function.

Fibromyalgia Power Food—These recipes use ingredients that can offer relief from fibromyalgia symptoms, like pain and fatigue.

Hashimoto's Power Food—These immune-boosting recipes use ingredients that can help protect your immune system and do not use ingredients that can aggravate Hashimoto's disease.

Hypoglycemia Power Food—These recipes are designed to help you control your blood sugar throughout the day and curb sugar cravings.

Insomnia—These recipes are designed with carefully selected ingredients to help you relax and improve your sleep.

Low-FODMAP for IBS—These recipes provide gut-healing foods and nutrients to help ease IBS symptoms.

Mood Booster—Although depression can't be cured with food, Mood Booster recipes use healthy whole foods that may help alleviate symptoms of depression.

Toxin Buster—These recipes contain ingredients that can help unload toxins accumulated in the body.

Tips

In addition to the labels, there are also helpful tips provided after each recipe. Let's look at the different types of tips each recipe can have:

A Closer Look—I will offer more information on a particular ingredient used in the recipe and how it contributes to healing your adrenal fatigue.

Prep Tip—I will offer you a prep tip that makes a recipe simpler and saves time.

Stretch Tip—I will walk you through how you can upcycle your meals, sides, and sauces to create something different.

Substitution Tip—I will provide substitutions for the ingredients that are not recommended for people with certain comorbidities. For a quick at-a-glance view, I also mark these ingredients in the ingredient list with these labels: [◆]IBS, [●]Hashimoto's, [▲]Toxin Overload, and [■]Fibromyalgia.

Too Tired to Cook—These tips switch the recipe up so that either it takes less than 10 minutes to cook and prepare or no cooking is required.

A note about shortcuts: If your busy lifestyle is a barrier to cooking, I urge you to take shortcuts to make things easier on yourself. Use pre-washed, precut, or frozen produce to save time, and prepare meals in bulk to freeze for later. Many of my busy clients pick one day to prepare meals for the whole week.

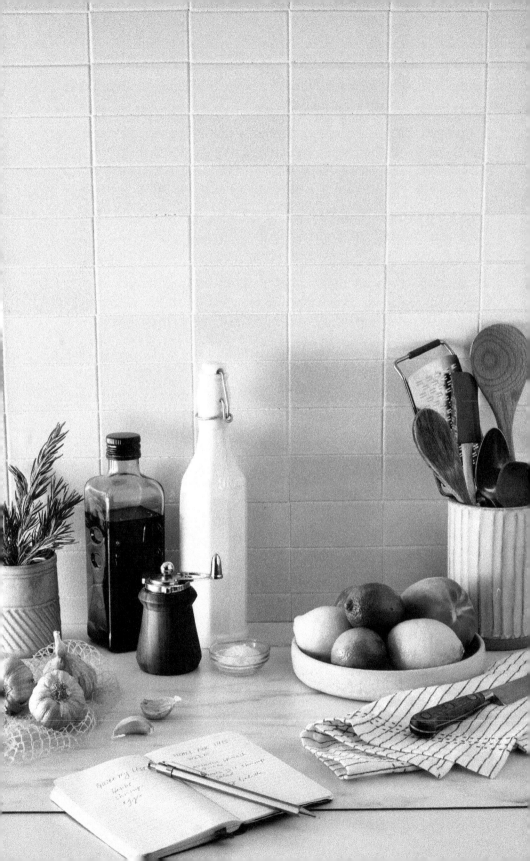

Chapter 3

The Meal Plans

Now that you understand the physiological backdrop to adrenal fatigue, I'm going to walk you through meal plans designed to help alleviate your symptoms. When it comes to making lasting changes, I'm a firm believer in taking baby steps. Before you begin your Week 1 plan, you will have a primer week to help you ease into new ways of eating.

When you make sudden changes to your diet, you may feel deprived of your favorite go-to foods, making it difficult to stick to the changes. I've included the primer week to help ease this transition.

The primer week is all about assessing your present lifestyle and eating habits and setting new intentions. Elimination of foods does not begin until Week 1. In addition to the four weekly meal plans, I have included an additional Flare-Up Meal Plan and guidelines on how to use it to navigate restaurant menus, travel, holidays, birthdays, and social events.

Primer Week

Making changes should not feel forced or like an obligation. Think about an event you dread attending—you'll always look for reasons not to go. Diet and lifestyle changes are the same way.

For the primer week, spend some time setting intentions for yourself. Write the intentions down on paper and keep the paper somewhere you can see it. Why does this change in your diet matter to you? Think about times when you've felt energetic and vibrant—what would it mean to feel that way again? Then, I want you to think about your day. What do you do on a daily basis out of habit and routine? For example:

* Stop at your regular coffee shop to pick up coffee every morning
* Make frequent stops at your work snack cabinet or vending machine
* Go for a walk midday to grab a drink, snack, or both
* Sit in front of the TV and order takeout for dinner
* Have a drink or two before or with dinner
* Watch TV in bed until you can fall asleep

These may seem like normal, harmless parts of your daily routine, but they can all have a negative impact on your adrenal glands. Relying heavily on processed snacks and meals for nourishment can decrease nutrient intake and increase inflammation. Meanwhile, excessive caffeine and screen time can increase cortisol levels.

When I help address my clients' negative habits related to food, I ask them to write down their daily schedules in detail and pinpoint habits that can be changed. When you decide for yourself what kind of changes you want to make, you are likely to stick with your plan longer.

A few things I want you to think about in your primer week are:

Water—Women should consume about 11 cups (2.7 liters), and men should consume about 16 cups (3.7 liters) of fluid per day, including water, food, and other sources of fluid (unless you have medical reasons to restrict fluid intake).

Sleep—Get seven to eight hours of uninterrupted sleep. Go to bed earlier to allow yourself time to unwind.

Rest—Reduce screen time (especially before bed) and take a five- to ten-minute rest break during the day whenever possible.

Food—Replace processed foods with whole foods. Drink unflavored sparkling water instead of soda. Snack on nuts instead of chips.

Coffee—Slowly reduce coffee intake by replacing it with decaffeinated coffee, water, or naturally decaffeinated teas (such as mint, chamomile, cinnamon, and lemon-ginger).

Alcohol—Start cutting back in all areas, both at home and at social events.

If you only follow half of the guidelines in the first week, that's okay. Rather than quitting because you think you have failed, congratulate yourself for what you have done, and continue toward your goal. Stay positive and visualize your success.

Week 1

On this meal plan, many meals are upcycled or repeated to reduce time spent in the kitchen. I provide a list after each week's meal plan on which foods to prepare in advance.

This week, you will eliminate a third of the foods on the "avoid" list: red meats (like pork, beef, duck, veal, and lamb), processed foods (like chips and sugary snack bars), and your personal symptom trigger foods. We won't completely eliminate sugar just yet, but we'll use limited amounts of maple syrup as opposed to artificial sugar substitutes. When grocery shopping, always try to purchase the best produce you can afford—quality impacts nutrient content.

Shopping List

Pantry

- Almond butter, unsalted (⅓ cup) (for IBS, substitute peanut butter)
- Baking powder, aluminum-free (¼ teaspoon)
- Baking soda (¼ teaspoon)
- Beans, black, unsalted, 1 (15-ounce) can
- Broth, chicken, unsalted (3 quarts)
- Brown rice pasta (3 cups cooked)
- Cashew butter, unsalted (2 tablespoons) (for IBS, substitute peanut butter)
- Chia seeds (5 tablespoons)
- Chickpeas, unsalted, 2 (15-ounce) cans
- Cocoa powder, unsweetened (1 teaspoon)
- Coconut aminos (¼ cup)
- Coconut water (1½ cups)
- Coriander, ground (1 tablespoon)
- Cumin, ground (3 tablespoons)
- Herbes de Provence (1 tablespoon)
- Maple syrup, pure (½ cup)
- Mustard, Dijon (2 tablespoons)
- Oats, rolled, gluten-free (½ cup)
- Oil, olive
- Oil, toasted sesame (2 tablespoons)
- Peppercorns, black
- Quinoa (2 cups uncooked)
- Rice, brown (4 cups cooked)
- Salt, kosher
- Tomato sauce (3½ cups) (omit for Hashimoto's)
- Tomatoes, crushed, 1 (15-ounce) can (omit for Hashimoto's)
- Tomatoes, diced, unsalted, 1 (16-ounce) can (omit for Hashimoto's)

- Vanilla extract, alcohol- and sugar-free (1 tablespoon)
- Vinegar, Champagne (1½ cups)
- Vinegar, sherry (¼ cup)
- Walnuts, chopped (1 tablespoon)

Produce
- Arugula, baby (3 cups)
- Asparagus (1 bunch)
- Avocado (1)
- Basil, fresh (1 bunch)
- Bean sprouts (2 cups)
- Bell pepper (1) (omit for Hashimoto's)
- Berries, fresh (your choice) (6⅓ cups)
- Cilantro, fresh (2 bunches)
- Eggplant (1 large) (omit for Hashimoto's)
- Garlic (1 or 2 heads) (for IBS, substitute garlic-infused oil or the green portions of 2 bunches scallions)
- Ginger, fresh, 1 (3-inch) piece
- Limes (2)
- Mint, fresh (1 bunch)
- Mushrooms, button, 1 (4-ounce) container
- Mushrooms, portabella (2) (for IBS, substitute oyster mushrooms)
- Onions, red (2) (for IBS, substitute the green portions of 1 bunch scallions)
- Onions, yellow (2) (for IBS, substitute the green portions of 1 bunch scallions)
- Parsley, fresh (1 bunch)
- Pineapple, chunks, fresh or frozen (1½ cups)
- Radishes (4)
- Scallions (1 bunch)
- Shallots, small to medium (5) (for IBS, substitute the green portions of 3 bunches scallions)
- Spinach, baby (5 cups, packed)
- Squash, delicata (1 large) (for IBS, substitute kabocha squash)
- Tomatoes, roma (5) or cherry (1 pint) (omit for Hashimoto's)
- Zucchini, medium (6)
- Zucchini, spiralized (4 cups)

Protein, Poultry, Fish, and Eggs
- Chicken, boneless, skinless breasts (2)
- Chicken, boneless, skinless thighs (1 pound)
- Eggs, large, cage-free, pasture-raised (15)
- Milk, plant-based, unsweetened (1 cup, for IBS, choose oat milk)
- Salmon, wild Atlantic (1½ pounds)
- Turkey, ground (1 pound)

Week 1 Meal Plan

DAY	SUNDAY	MONDAY	TUESDAY
BREAKFAST	Uplift Green Smoothie (page 75)	2 hard-boiled eggs 1 cup fresh berries	2 hard-boiled eggs 1 cup fresh berries
LUNCH	One-Pot Chicken and Quinoa* (page 83)	Leftover One-Pot Chicken and Quinoa	Leftover Best Turkey Burgers
SNACK	1 cup fresh berries	Flourless Chickpea Blondies* (page 139)	Leftover Flourless Chickpea Blondies
DINNER	Sautéed Mushroom and Quinoa Bowl (page 100)	Best Turkey Burgers* (page 117)	Roasted Eggplant Ragù with brown rice pasta* (page 119)

WEDNESDAY	THURSDAY	FRIDAY	SATURDAY
Uplift Green Smoothie (page 75)	2 hard-boiled eggs 1 cup fresh berries	Uplift Green Smoothie (page 75)	Creamy Chocolate Oatmeal (page 74)
Leftover Roasted Eggplant Ragù with brown rice pasta	Leftover Baked Mustard Salmon with Leftover Roasted Summer Vegetables	Leftover Roasted Vegetable Fried Rice	Shakshuka (page 80)
1 cup fresh berries	Leftover Flourless Chickpea Blondies	1 cup fresh berries	Leftover Flourless Chickpea Blondies
Baked Mustard Salmon* (page 116) with Roasted Summer Vegetables* (page 131)	Roasted Vegetable Fried Rice* (page 96)	30-Minute Chicken Pho (page 112)	Roasted Vegetable Grain Bowl (page 90)

Prepare in advance: 6 hard-boiled eggs, 3 cups cooked brown rice pasta, 4 cups cooked brown rice, Flourless Chickpea Blondies (page 139)

*The recipes with asterisks are ones that will be used again. If you need more than four to six servings of one of these recipes, make more!

Week 2

This week, let's try to eliminate the next third of "avoid" foods: corn, soy, and dairy products. When preparing the meals, think about what worked and didn't work for you in Week 1. It's also important for you to think about how you are managing your day-to-day stress, hydration needs, and sleep.

Shopping List

Pantry

- Baking powder, aluminum-free (1 teaspoon)
- Baking soda (½ teaspoon)
- Beans, black, unsalted, 1 (15-ounce) can
- Broth, unsalted chicken or vegetable (2 quarts)
- Cashew butter, unsalted (1¼ cups) (for IBS, substitute peanut butter)
- Cashews, raw, unsalted (1 cup)
- Chia seeds (1½ cups)
- Chickpeas, unsalted, 1 (15-ounce) can
- Cinnamon, ground (1 teaspoon)
- Cocoa powder, unsweetened (⅔ cup)
- Coconut water (1 cup)
- Coriander, ground (2 tablespoons)
- Cumin, ground (1 tablespoon)
- Cumin seeds (1 tablespoon)
- Flaxseed (1 cup)
- Flour, almond (1 cup) (for IBS, substitute oat flour)
- Flour, buckwheat (1 cup)
- Garam masala (1½ teaspoons)
- Garlic powder (2 teaspoons) (omit for IBS)
- Lentils, dried, red (2 cups)
- Maple syrup, pure (¾ cup)
- Mustard, Dijon (3 tablespoons)
- Nuts, roasted, unsalted, your choice (¼ cup chopped)
- Oats, rolled, gluten-free (4 cups)
- Oil, coconut (1 cup)
- Oil, olive
- Pecans, unsalted (1 cup chopped)
- Pepitas (pumpkin seeds), unsalted (½ cup)
- Peppercorns, black
- Pine nuts, unsalted (¼ cup)
- Potato starch (1 cup) (for Hashimoto's, substitute almond flour)
- Quinoa (4 cups cooked)
- Raisins (2 tablespoons)
- Rice, brown (4 cups cooked)
- Salt, coarse sea (1 teaspoon), such as Maldon sea salt flakes
- Salt, kosher
- Sesame seeds (½ cup)
- Stock, unsalted chicken (1 quart)
- Sumac (1 teaspoon)
- Tahini (2 tablespoons)

- Tomato paste (3 tablespoons) (omit for Hashimoto's)
- Tomato sauce, 1 (15-ounce) can (omit for Hashimoto's)
- Turmeric, ground (4 teaspoons)
- Vanilla beans (¼ teaspoon), optional
- Vanilla extract, alcohol- and sugar-free (1½ teaspoons)
- Vinegar, apple cider (2 tablespoons)
- Vinegar, Champagne (1½ cups)
- Vinegar, sherry (2 tablespoons)

Produce
- Arugula, baby (4 cups)
- Avocado (1)
- Berries, fresh (your choice) (5 cups)
- Blueberries, frozen (1½ cups)
- Broccoli (1 head)
- Celery (2 stalks)
- Chard, rainbow (1 bunch)
- Cilantro, fresh (1 or 2 bunches)
- Cucumbers, seedless (2)
- Garlic (1 head) (for IBS, replace with garlic-infused olive oil or the green portions of 1 bunch scallions)
- Ginger, fresh, 1 (4-inch) piece
- Lemons (2)
- Lettuce, butter (2 heads)
- Limes (2)
- Onion, yellow (1) (for IBS, replace with the green portions of 3 bunches scallions)
- Onions, red (2) (for IBS, replace with the green portions of 3 bunches scallions)
- Parsley, fresh (1 or 2 bunches)
- Pineapple, chunks, fresh or frozen (1 cup)
- Radishes (5)
- Shallots, small to medium (5) (for IBS, replace with the green portions of 1 bunch scallions)
- Spinach, baby (6 cups)
- Tomatoes, cherry (2 cups) (omit for Hashimoto's)
- Tomatoes, medium (2) (omit for Hashimoto's)
- Zucchini, medium (1)

Protein, Poultry, Fish, and Eggs
- Chicken, boneless, skinless breasts (1½ pounds)
- Chicken, boneless, skinless thighs (1 pound)
- Chicken, tenders (1 pound)
- Eggs, large, cage-free, pasture-raised (5)
- Milk, plant-based, unsweetened (¾ cup, for IBS, choose oat milk)
- Salmon, wild Atlantic (1½ pounds)
- Shrimp, wild, peeled, and deveined (1½ pounds)
- Yogurt, coconut, unsweetened (½ cup)

Week 2 Meal Plan

DAY	SUNDAY	MONDAY	TUESDAY
BREAKFAST	Connor's "Cereal" Granola* (page 71) with Creamy Vanilla Cashew Milk* (page 148)	Leftover Connor's "Cereal" Granola with Leftover Creamy Vanilla Cashew Milk	Leftover Connor's "Cereal" Granola with Leftover Creamy Vanilla Cashew Milk
LUNCH	Quinoa and Arugula Salad with Vegetables* (page 82)	Leftover Quinoa and Arugula Salad with Vegetables	Leftover Simple Base Salad with 2 hard-boiled eggs
SNACK	Cashew Butter Cups* (page 137)	1 cup fresh berries	1 cup fresh berries
DINNER	Chicken Tikka Masala Grain Bowl* (page 94)	Leftover Chicken Tikka Masala Grain Bowl with Simple Base Salad* (page 133)	Shrimp Tacos with Black Bean Salad* (page 121)

WEDNESDAY	THURSDAY	FRIDAY	SATURDAY
Leftover Connor's "Cereal" Granola with Leftover Creamy Vanilla Cashew Milk	Uplift Green Smoothie (page 75)	Uplift Green Smoothie (page 75)	Fluffiest Raspberry Pancakes (page 72)
Leftover Shrimp Tacos with Black Bean Salad	Leftover Connor's Chicken Soup	Leftover Creamy Masoor Dal Grain Bowl	Leftover Baked Mustard Salmon with Leftover Sautéed Broccoli with Raisins
1 cup fresh berries	Leftover Cashew Butter Cups	Leftover Cashew Butter Cups	Leftover Cashew Butter Cups
Connor's Chicken Soup* (page 104)	Creamy Masoor Dal Grain Bowl* (page 92)	Baked Mustard Salmon* (page 116) with Sautéed Broccoli with Raisins* (page 130)	Crispy Chicken Tenders (page 123)

Prepare in advance: 4 cups cooked quinoa, 4 cups cooked brown rice, 2 hard-boiled eggs, Connor's "Cereal" Granola (page 71), Creamy Vanilla Cashew Milk (page 148), Cashew Butter Cups (page 137)

*The recipes with asterisks are ones that will be used again. If you need more than four to six servings of one of these recipes, make more!

Week 3

After two weeks of following the plan, you likely have a good sense of how the diet works. This week, you'll eliminate the final third of the "avoid" foods: gluten and all added sugar. (None of the recipes in this book contains gluten.) By now, you may have a favorite recipe that you want to make again. If you decide to make changes to this week's meal plan, you can choose any recipes as long as they don't use maple syrup—or, if the recipe you choose does use maple syrup, remove it (or replace it with dates). Remember to continue eliminating any of your personal trigger foods!

Shopping List

Pantry

- Almond butter, unsalted (6 tablespoons) (for IBS, substitute peanut butter)
- Baking soda (1 teaspoon)
- Beans, black, unsalted, 1 (15-ounce) can
- Bread crumbs, chickpea or gluten-free (⅓ cup)
- Broth, chicken, unsalted (2 quarts) (or make 1 batch Chicken Bone Broth, page 106)
- Cashew butter, unsalted (1 tablespoon) (for IBS, substitute peanut butter)
- Chia seeds (1¾ cups)
- Chickpeas, unsalted, 1 (15-ounce) can
- Cinnamon, ground (2 teaspoons)
- Cocoa powder, unsweetened (2 tablespoons)
- Coconut aminos (2 tablespoons)
- Coconut water (1 cup)
- Cumin, ground (2 tablespoons)
- Flaxseed (1 cup)
- Flour, almond (3½ cups) (for IBS, substitute gluten-free oat flour)
- Flour, oat, gluten-free (1 cup)
- Garlic powder (2 teaspoons) (omit for IBS)
- Hemp seeds (1 tablespoon), optional
- Mustard, Dijon (3 tablespoons)
- Oats, rolled, gluten-free (1 cup)
- Oil, olive
- Peppercorns, black
- Pine nuts, unsalted (¼ cup)
- Potato starch (1 cup) (for Hashimoto's, substitute almond flour)
- Quinoa (4 cups cooked)
- Rice, brown (1 cup cooked)
- Salt, kosher
- Sesame seeds (½ cup)
- Stock, chicken, unsalted (1 quart)

- Vanilla beans
  (¼ teaspoon), optional
- Vanilla extract, alcohol- and
  sugar-free (1 tablespoon)

- Vinegar, sherry (½ cup)
- Walnuts, unsalted (1 cup)

Produce

- Apples, Fuji (2 or 3)
- Arugula, baby (8 cups)
- Bananas (1 or 2)
- Basil, fresh (2 bunches)
- Bean sprouts (2 cups)
- Bell pepper (1) (omit
  for Hashimoto's)
- Berries, fresh (your choice)
  (2 cups)
- Chard, rainbow (1 bunch)
- Cilantro, fresh (2 bunches)
- Cucumbers, seedless (2)
- Dates, medjool (6)
- Garlic (1 head) (for IBS,
  substitute garlic-infused
  oil or the green portions of
  1 bunch scallions)
- Ginger, fresh, 1 (2-inch) piece
- Limes (2)
- Mint, fresh (1 bunch)
- Mushrooms, portabella
  (2) (for IBS, replace with
  oyster mushrooms)

- Onion (1) (for IBS, substi-
  tute the green portions of
  1 bunch scallions)
- Parsley, fresh (1 bunch)
- Pineapple, chunks, fresh or
  frozen (1 cup)
- Radishes (5)
- Scallions (1 bunch)
- Shallots, small to medium (4)
  (for IBS, substitute the green
  portions of 1 bunch scallions)
- Spinach, baby (6 cups)
- Squash, butternut, spiralized,
  (1 cup) (for IBS, substitute
  spiralized zucchini)
- Tomatoes, cherry (2 cups)
  (omit for Hashimoto's)
- Zucchini, medium (2)
- Zucchini, spiralized (4 cups)

Poultry, Fish, and Eggs

- Chicken, boneless,
  skinless breasts (2)
- Chicken, tenders (1 pound)
- Eggs, large, cage-free,
  pasture-raised (12)

- Salmon, wild Atlantic
  (1½ pounds)
- Turkey, ground (1½ pounds)

Week 3 Meal Plan

DAY	SUNDAY	MONDAY	TUESDAY
BREAKFAST	Butternut Squash Nest Eggs* (page 68)	Apple-Chia Power Muffins* (page 69)	Leftover Apple-Chia Power Muffins
LUNCH	Quinoa and Arugula Salad with Vegetables* (page 82)	Leftover Best Turkey Burgers with Leftover Quinoa and Arugula Salad with Vegetables	Leftover Lazy Day Italian Wedding Soup
SNACK	Chocolate Energy Bites* (page 136)	Leftover Chocolate Energy Bites	Leftover Chocolate Energy Bites
DINNER	Best Turkey Burgers* (page 117)	Lazy Day Italian Wedding Soup* (page 109)	Baked Mustard Salmon* (page 116) with Simple Base Salad* (page 133)

WEDNESDAY	THURSDAY	FRIDAY	SATURDAY
Leftover Butternut Squash Nest Eggs	Uplift Green Smoothie (page 75)	Leftover Apple-Chia Power Muffins	Uplift Green Smoothie (page 75)
Leftover Baked Mustard Salmon with Leftover Simple Base Salad	Leftover 30-Minute Chicken Pho	Leftover Crispy Chicken Tenders	Leftover Sautéed Mushroom and Quinoa Bowl
1 cup fresh berries	Leftover Chocolate Energy Bites	Leftover Chocolate Energy Bites	1 cup fresh berries
30-Minute Chicken Pho* (page 112)	Crispy Chicken Tenders* (page 123)	Sautéed Mushroom and Quinoa Bowl* (page 100)	Hearty Black Bean Burgers (page 86)

Prepare in advance: 4 cups cooked quinoa, 1 cup cooked brown rice, Apple-Chia Power Muffins (page 69), Chocolate Energy Bites (page 136), Optional: Chicken Bone Broth (page 106; otherwise buy store-bought broth)

*The recipes with asterisks are ones that will be used again. If you need more than four to six servings of one of these recipes, make more!

Week 4

Congratulations! You have completely eliminated all the foods on the "avoid" list. Going forward, I encourage you to continue leaving out these foods. By this point, you should start to feel the effects of the adrenal fatigue diet—you may have more energy, fewer gastrointestinal symptoms, and less brain fog.

After this week, you can create your own meals and meal plans. If you're thinking about reintroducing foods on the "avoid" list, I suggest doing so only after eight weeks or so. It takes time to see all the potential changes from this diet plan, and reintroducing common trigger foods too early will prevent you from experiencing the full benefits of those changes.

Shopping List

Pantry

- Bay leaves (2)
- Beans, black, unsalted, 3 (15-ounce) cans
- Beans, kidney, unsalted, 1 (15-ounce) can
- Broth, chicken or vegetable, unsalted (6 cups)
- Cashew butter, unsalted (2 tablespoons) (for IBS, substitute peanut butter)
- Chia seeds (½ cup)
- Chili powder (1 teaspoon) (omit for Hashimoto's)
- Cocoa powder, unsweetened (2 teaspoons)
- Coconut water (1½ cups)
- Coriander, ground (2 tablespoons)
- Cumin, ground (2 tablespoons)
- Cumin seeds (1 tablespoon)
- Lentils, green or brown, unsalted, 1 (15-ounce) can
- Lentils, red, dried (2 cups)
- Mustard, Dijon (3 tablespoons)
- Oats, rolled, gluten-free (1 cup)
- Oil, olive
- Oregano, dried (2 teaspoons)
- Peppercorns, black
- Pine nuts, unsalted (¼ cup) (or nuts or seeds of your choice)
- Quinoa (2 cups uncooked)
- Raisins (2 tablespoons)
- Salt, kosher
- Stock, vegetable, unsalted (1 quart)
- Sumac (1 teaspoon)
- Tahini (½ cup)
- Tomato paste (1 tablespoon)
- Tomato sauce (1½ cups) (for Hashimoto's, replace with chicken or vegetable broth)
- Tomatoes, roasted, unsalted, 1 (28-ounce) can
- Turmeric, ground (1½ teaspoons)
- Vinegar, Champagne (1½ cups)
- Vinegar, sherry (¼ cup)
- Walnuts, chopped (2 tablespoons)

Produce

- Arugula, baby (5 cups)
- Asparagus spears (8)
- Avocados (3)
- Beets, whole, precooked (5 to 7)
- Bell peppers (2) (omit for Hashimoto's)
- Berries, fresh (your choice), 1 (6-ounce) container
- Blueberries, frozen (1 cup)
- Broccoli (1 head)
- Cantaloupe (1)
- Carrots, baby (1 bag), to dip in Roasted Sweet Potato "Hummus"
- Cauliflower, florets, frozen (1 cup)
- Celery (1 bunch), to dip in Roasted Sweet Potato "Hummus"
- Cilantro, fresh (1 bunch)
- Cucumber, seedless (1)
- Date, medjool (1)
- Garlic (1 head) (for IBS, replace with garlic-infused olive oil or the green portions of 1 bunch scallions)
- Ginger, fresh, 1 (2-inch) piece
- Green beans, whole (1 cup, about 25 beans)
- Lemons (2)
- Lettuce, butter (2 heads)
- Limes (4)
- Mint, fresh (1 bunch)
- Onions, red (3) (for IBS, replace with the green portions of 3 bunches scallions)
- Orange, large (1)
- Parsley, fresh (1 bunch)
- Pineapple, chunks, fresh or frozen (½ cup)
- Radishes (6)
- Shallots, small to medium (6) (for IBS, replace with the green portions of 2 bunches scallions)
- Spinach, baby (5 cups)
- Sweet potatoes, large (3)
- Tomato, medium (1) (omit for Hashimoto's)
- Tomatoes, cherry (1 cup) (omit for Hashimoto's)
- Zucchini, medium (2)

Protein, Poultry, Fish, and Eggs

- Chicken, boneless, skinless thighs (1 pound)
- Eggs, large, cage-free, pasture-raised (12)
- Milk, plant-based, unsweetened (1 quart, for IBS, choose oat milk)
- Salmon, wild Atlantic (1½ pounds)
- Shrimp, wild, peeled and deveined (1½ pounds)

Week 4 Meal Plan

DAY	SUNDAY	MONDAY	TUESDAY
BREAKFAST	Creamy Chocolate Oatmeal (page 74)	Muffin Tin Frittatas* (page 76)	Leftover Muffin Tin Frittatas
LUNCH	Crunchy Summer Salad (page 85)	Leftover Roasted Vegetable Chili	Leftover Baked Mustard Salmon with Leftover Sautéed Broccoli with Raisins
SNACK	Nutty Blueberry Smoothie (page 143)	Roasted Sweet Potato "Hummus"* (page 129) with carrots and celery	Leftover Roasted Sweet Potato "Hummus" with carrots and celery
DINNER	Roasted Vegetable Chili* (page 110)	Baked Mustard Salmon* (page 116) with Sautéed Broccoli with Raisins* (page 130)	Warm Green Lentil Salad* (page 118)

WEDNESDAY	THURSDAY	FRIDAY	SATURDAY
Leftover Muffin Tin Frittatas	Leftover Muffin Tin Frittatas	Creamy Chocolate Oatmeal (page 74)	Uplift Green Smoothie (page 75)
Leftover Warm Green Lentil Salad	Leftover Roasted Beet Salad with Orange and Avocado	Leftover One-Pot Chicken and Quinoa	Leftover Creamy Masoor Dal Grain Bowl
Leftover Roasted Sweet Potato "Hummus" with carrots and celery	Leftover Roasted Sweet Potato "Hummus" with carrots and celery	Leftover Roasted Sweet Potato "Hummus" with carrots and celery	Coconut-Melon Cooler (page 141)
Roasted Beet Salad with Orange and Avocado* (page 132)	One-Pot Chicken and Quinoa* (page 83)	Creamy Masoor Dal Grain Bowl* (page 92)	Shrimp Tacos with Black Bean Salad (page 121)

Prepare in advance: 2 cups cooked quinoa, Muffin Tin Frittatas (page 76), Roasted Sweet Potato "Hummus" (page 129)

*The recipes with asterisks are ones that will be used again. If you need more than four to six servings of one of these recipes, make more!

The Flare-Up Meal Plan

A "flare-up" is what it sounds like—a sudden exacerbation of a medical condition. Adrenal fatigue flare-ups can happen due to illness, anxiety or stress, poor diet, and sleep deprivation, among other things. Regardless of the reason, if you are experiencing flare-ups, there are a few things I want you to focus on for this week: stress management, diet, and proper hydration.

Manage Your Stress—How are you currently managing your stress? What are your stress triggers? What has worked best for you in the past? Was it seeing a therapist? Working out more regularly? Meditating?

Eat Right—Are you drinking alcohol or caffeinated beverages? What foods (if any) have you reintroduced that are on the "avoid" list?

Stay Hydrated—Are you drinking enough water? How can you manage your water intake to ensure that you meet your body's daily fluid needs (see page 33)?

Shopping List

Pantry

- Baking powder, aluminum-free (1 teaspoon)
- Baking soda (½ teaspoon)
- Beans, black, unsalted, 1 (15-ounce) can
- Broth, chicken, unsalted (1⅓ cups)
- Chickpeas, unsalted, 1 (15-ounce) can
- Coconut aminos (2 tablespoons)
- Coriander, ground (2 tablespoons)
- Cumin, ground (2 tablespoons)
- Flour, buckwheat (1 cup)
- Lentils, green or brown, unsalted, 1 (15-ounce) can
- Mustard, Dijon (½ tablespoon)
- Nuts, raw or roasted and unsalted, for snacking, like walnuts, cashews, almonds, or peanuts (½ cup) (for IBS, choose peanuts)
- Oil, coconut (2 tablespoons, plus more for cooking)
- Oil, olive
- Oil, toasted sesame (2 tablespoons)
- Peppercorns, black
- Pine nuts (⅛ cup)
- Quinoa (2 cups uncooked)
- Rice, brown (4 cups cooked)
- Salt, kosher
- Stock, chicken or vegetable, unsalted (3 cups)

- Tomato sauce, 1 (16-ounce) can (for Hashimoto's, substitute chicken or vegetable broth)
- Tomatoes, diced, unsalted, 1 (16-ounce) can (omit for Hashimoto's)
- Vinegar, apple cider (2 tablespoons)
- Vinegar, Champagne (1½ cups)
- Vinegar, sherry (½ cup)

Produce

- Arugula, baby (10 cups)
- Asparagus spears (5)
- Avocados (2)
- Bananas (3 or 4)
- Beets, whole, precooked (5 to 7)
- Bell pepper (1) (omit for Hashimoto's)
- Berries, fresh (your choice) (3½ cups)
- Blueberries, frozen (1½ cups)
- Cilantro, fresh (1 bunch)
- Garlic (1 head) (for IBS, replace with garlic-infused olive oil or the green portions of 1 bunch scallions)
- Ginger, fresh, 1 (4-inch) piece
- Mint, fresh (1 bunch)
- Mushrooms, portabella (2) (for IBS, replace with oyster mushrooms)
- Onion, red (1) (for IBS, replace with the green portions of 1 bunch scallions)
- Onion, yellow (1) (for IBS, replace with the green portions of 1 bunch scallions)
- Orange, large (1)
- Parsley, fresh (1 bunch)
- Radishes (4)
- Shallots, small to medium (4) (for IBS, replace with the green portions of 1 bunch scallions)
- Spinach, baby (2 cups)
- Squash, butternut, spiralized (2 cups) (for IBS, replace with 2 medium zucchini)
- Squash, kabocha, medium (1)
- Strawberries, frozen (3 cups)
- Vegetables, mixed, your choice (1 cup)
- Zucchini, medium (2)

Protein, Poultry, and Eggs

- Chicken, boneless, skinless thighs (1 pound)
- Eggs, cage-free, pasture-raised (23)
- Milk, plant-based, unsweetened (¾ cup, for IBS, choose oat milk)

The Flare-Up Meal Plan

DAY	SUNDAY	MONDAY	TUESDAY
BREAKFAST	Fluffiest Raspberry Pancakes* (page 72)	2 hard-boiled eggs with ½ cup fresh berries	2 hard-boiled eggs with ½ cup fresh berries
LUNCH	Shakshuka (page 80)	Leftover Kabocha Squash Soup	Leftover Roasted Vegetable Grain Bowl
SNACK	Strawberry-Banana Nice Cream (page 138)	2 tablespoons roasted, unsalted nuts	2 tablespoons roasted, unsalted nuts
DINNER	Kabocha Squash Soup* (page 108)	Roasted Vegetable Grain Bowl* (page 90)	Warm Green Lentil Salad* (page 118)

WEDNESDAY	THURSDAY	FRIDAY	SATURDAY
2 hard-boiled eggs with ½ cup fresh berries	Butternut Squash Nest Eggs (page 68)	Butternut Squash Nest Eggs (page 68)	Leftover Fluffiest Raspberry Pancakes
Leftover Warm Green Lentil Salad	Leftover Roasted Vegetable Fried Rice	Leftover Roasted Beet Salad with Orange and Avocado	Leftover One-Pot Chicken and Quinoa
2 tablespoons roasted, unsalted nuts	1 cup fresh berries	1 cup fresh berries	Strawberry-Banana Nice Cream (page 138)
Roasted Vegetable Fried Rice* (page 96)	Roasted Beet Salad with Orange and Avocado* (page 132)	One-Pot Chicken and Quinoa* (page 83)	Sautéed Mushroom and Quinoa Bowl (page 100)

Prepare in advance: 6 hard-boiled eggs, 2½ cups cooked quinoa, 4 cups cooked brown rice

*The recipes with asterisks are ones that will be used again. If you need more than four to six servings of one of these recipes, make more!

Build Your Own Maintenance Plans

This book provides you with detailed, step-by-step weekly meal plans, but you don't have to follow them to a T. After browsing the recipes in part 2 of this book, you may feel motivated to create your own meal plan (blank pages for meal planning are on page 62). I strongly encourage you to design meal plans that cater to your own lifestyle. When planning your own menu, here are a few things to keep in mind.

1. Be mindful of the ingredients in your weekly menu. You don't want to end up with an excessively long grocery list and lots of unused food. For example, if zucchini is on the menu one day, look for another recipe that includes them so you don't end up with leftover zucchini and nothing to cook with it.

2. Think about how you can make your meals more balanced, without overusing animal protein or carbohydrates. For example, if you had a carbohydrate-heavy lunch (like Creamy Masoor Dal Grain Bowl, page 92), choose a recipe that uses mostly protein and vegetables (like 30-Minute Chicken Pho, page 112) for dinner.

3. Eat mindfully. Our eating habits often reflect our stress levels—poor stress management can lead to poor nutrition. For example, if you have a stressful day at work, you might seek out unhealthy comfort food and drinks after work. It's important to be aware of the relationship between stress and food so that we can plan with it in mind.

4. Pay attention to your emotions (sadness, boredom, stress, anxiety, avoidance, frustration, etc.). When you feel the urge to turn to your guilty pleasure food or if you find yourself overeating, stop and ask yourself why you want and need this food. Are you truly hungry? (And if so, can you make modifications to the meal to make it nutritious?) Or are you thirsty, tired, or feeling bad? I suggest you make a list of things other than comfort food that make you feel happy, comfortable, relaxed, and satisfied. Whenever you feel like your emotions are controlling your relationship with food, refer back to that list to help you avoid negative decisions around eating.

Mindful eating cannot be perfected overnight. My clients and I often work on emotional eating for months before they start to reconnect with their bodies' needs. Paying more attention to your hunger, satiation, and emotions can reduce emotional and binge eating habits and allow you to address your feelings in a positive way.

Life Beyond the Meal Plan

Congratulations on completing the four-week meal plan! By following the plan consistently, you have become more comfortable in the kitchen and created invaluable lifestyle habits that will last. You've trained your palate to enjoy more wholesome, fresh, nutritious foods. As you explore life beyond the meal plan, remember that when you reintroduce old diet and lifestyle habits, your risk of flare-ups increases. If a flare-up does occur, you can always turn to the Flare-Up Meal Plan (page 50). In this section, I'll walk you through tips and strategies on how to maintain the diet and continue enjoying life as you transition into the maintenance stage.

Restaurants

You have to consider diet and lifestyle as a combined unit in order to make positive changes for your health. You can't put your life on hold while you make these changes—and you shouldn't. Once you understand the building blocks of the adrenal fatigue diet, it is fairly easy to navigate restaurants and events. Here are a few things to keep in mind:

* Most restaurants will offer something that meets adrenal fatigue diet guidelines. Think beyond entrées and explore appetizers and side menus.
* Don't be shy about requesting substitutions in dishes when you go out to eat. Many restaurants are more than willing to accommodate diet restrictions.
* It may be impossible to strictly follow dietary guidelines when you go to someone else's house for dinner, and that's okay—just return to your routine with the next meal.

Strategies for Dining Out

TYPE OF FOOD	AVOID/LIMIT	BETTER CHOICES
ASIAN	Avoid brown-colored sauces, which are likely to contain refined sugar and soy sauce. Thai restaurants often use refined sugar in fried rice or noodles, so always ask whether the sauce contains soy sauce or sugar. Avoid sugar, gluten, and soy sauce (which contains gluten).	Request gluten-free soy sauce (also known as tamari). Look for menu items that are sautéed with garlic and ginger (if you have IBS, avoid garlic). Look for rice, soups, and sautéed dishes that are composed of rice (white or brown), lean protein, and vegetables. Examples:* Chinese: chicken and broccoli with brown rice Thai: papaya salad, chicken satay, steamed whole fish Japanese: sushi or sashimi, seaweed salad, green salad Vietnamese: chicken or vegetable pho with rice noodles (if the noodles are gluten-free and the broth is sugar-free), chicken or fish with rice and vegetables, spring or summer rolls (if the wrapper is gluten-free) *Always ask for no soy sauce or sugar added.

TYPE OF FOOD	AVOID/LIMIT	BETTER CHOICES
MEXICAN	Avoid corn or wheat flour and cheese.	Order guacamole with fresh vegetables (rather than fried chips) for dipping. Look for taco lettuce wraps, lean protein bowls, or entrée salads with rice, beans, and guacamole. Try stuffed bell peppers with rice and a protein (but avoid bell peppers if you have Hashimoto's).
ITALIAN	Avoid gluten and dairy (like in pastas with cheese).	Look for gluten-free pasta options (they are fairly easy to find nowadays). Look for pasta with vegetables or lean protein, with either pesto or tomato sauce, and skip the cheese. (If you have Hashimoto's, avoid tomatoes.) Choose a grilled or broiled protein with vegetables. Choose soup or salad (check the starters and sides section of the menu).

Strategies for Dining Out

TYPE OF FOOD	AVOID/LIMIT	BETTER CHOICES
MEDITERRANEAN	Avoid gluten (like pita bread) and dairy (like Halloumi and feta cheese).	Look for grilled lean protein with vegetables. Choose sautéed vegetable sides and salads.
AMERICAN	Avoid gluten, dairy, red meats, heavy or fried foods (such as hamburgers, pizza, and pasta), and condiments with lots of sugar (like ketchup and Worcestershire sauce).	Include vegetable-based appetizers and sides. Your main dish should have a lean protein (chicken, fish, turkey, or beans) with whole, gluten-free grains, starchy vegetables (like sweet potato), or other non-starchy vegetables. Use oil and vinegar as condiments.

TYPE OF FOOD	AVOID/LIMIT	BETTER CHOICES
BUFFET	In general, avoid heavily dressed foods. Look for dishes that use simple, whole ingredients. Avoid highly processed condiments, like mayonnaise and syrup.	Browse the buffet section before making up your plate. Look for lean protein, vegetables, fresh fruits, and gluten-free options. For condiments and dressings, look for fresh fruits, oils, and vinegars. Examples: Vegetable omelet with avocado and fresh berries Salad with lean protein and non-starchy vegetables Grilled or broiled protein with gluten-free grains and roasted vegetables
DESSERT	Limit and then eliminate added sugar and dairy. (For Week 1, choose a dessert that is low in sugar and dairy.)	Choose sorbet instead of ice cream and fruit crumbles rather than cake. Starting in Weeks 2 and 3, try to choose fresh fruits and nuts for dessert. (More delicious dessert options are in chapter 10 on page 135.)

Celebrations

Many of my clients say that holidays can be a source of anxiety when following a meal plan—but if you come in prepared, there's nothing to worry about. Here are a few tips on how to navigate the holidays.

Be open about your alcohol consumption—Don't be shy about letting people know you're not drinking alcohol. If you want to feel included, order a club soda. If you decide to drink alcohol, limit consumption to recommended guidelines (up to one drink per day for women and up to two drinks per day for men) and consume a large glass of water for every drink.

Eat simpler desserts—Choose a fresh fruit–based dessert rather than a heavy, sugary dessert made with highly processed ingredients. Stick to small portions.

Be prepared—Study the menu before you go and preselect your food so you already know what you can have. If it's a buffet, browse all the food options before you begin filling your plate.

Never go hungry—If dinner is not until eight o'clock and you feel hungry at six, eat a high-fiber, high-protein snack, such as a handful of nuts with berries.

Travel

Vacations shouldn't be stressful, so I make sure to meet with my clients before they travel to address their anxiety over eating while traveling and help them stay prepared. Here is some guidance to get you through the airport and your destination.

Airport: There are lots of fast food options or highly processed snacks at the airport. Make sure you bring the following items with you:

※ An empty water bottle to fill up after you go through airport security
※ Gluten-free instant oatmeal packets
※ Single-serve nut butter packets (unsalted, no sugar or oil added)
※ Raw or roasted unsalted nuts
※ Naturally caffeine-free tea

* Snack bars with simple, whole ingredients (no added sugar or preservatives)
* Gluten-free seed crackers
* Fruits that travel well, like apples and pears

Destination: If you know where you will be dining, review the menus in advance. If you need to substitute menu items, choose lean protein, vegetables, and fresh fruits.

Come Back for a Refresh

If you stray from the plan, jump right back in where you left off. Don't write off all your progress just because you had a glass of wine. Reread the intentions you wrote down at the beginning of your journey, and remind yourself why you began the diet. If necessary, start over with Week 1 and make your way through back to Week 4.

Here are ways to combat common challenges:

If you're returning from vacation, where you overindulged—Leave any guilt or shame at the door, and start again with Week 1 of the plan. Accepting a fresh start will help you move forward rather than continuing to eat the same way you did on vacation.

If you're busy with work and it's tough to cook meals—Rather than putting the adrenal fatigue diet on hold, review the meal plan for the current week you are on and see whether you can choose simple meals that are similar to these recipes. Reread the Foods to Avoid and Healing Foods lists in chapter 2 (page 20) and follow the guidelines as best you can.

If you're so stressed with work and life, and you just want to order takeout and watch a movie—I hear this often. If you decide to order takeout, adhere to the Foods to Avoid and Healing Foods lists as much as you can. To avoid overeating, practice mindful eating: Try eating first and then watching a movie or TV show, rather than watching while you eat.

Create Your Own Meal Plan

DAY	SUNDAY	MONDAY	TUESDAY
BREAKFAST			
LUNCH			
SNACK			
DINNER			

WEDNESDAY	THURSDAY	FRIDAY	SATURDAY

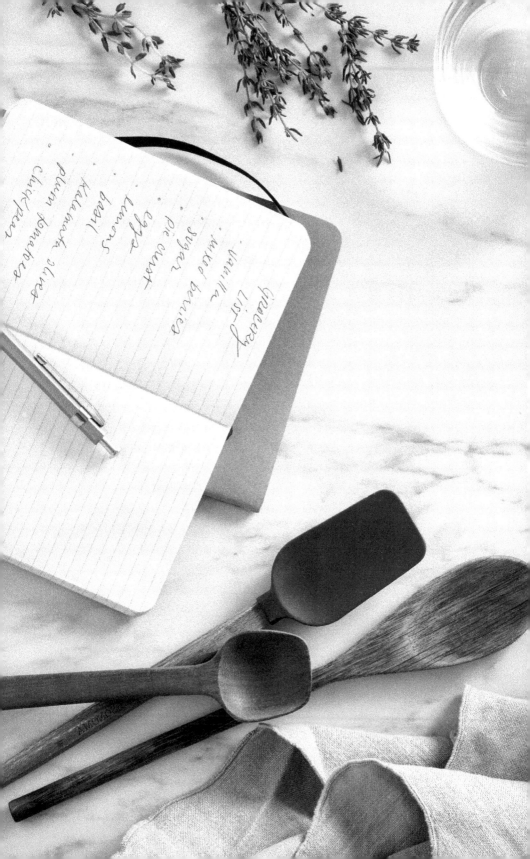

Grocery List

- mixed berries
- vanilla
- pie crust
- sugar
- eggs
- lemons
- basil
- Kalamata olives
- plum tomatoes
- chickpeas

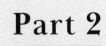

Part 2

The Recipes

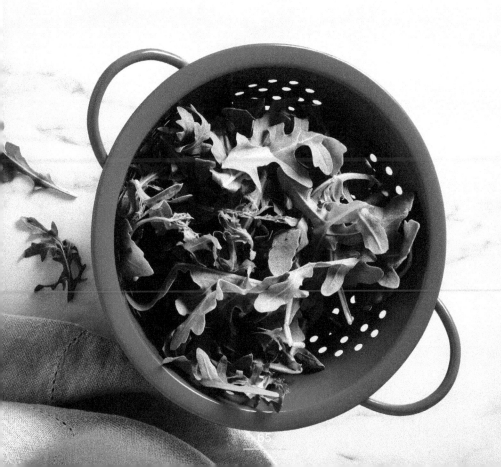

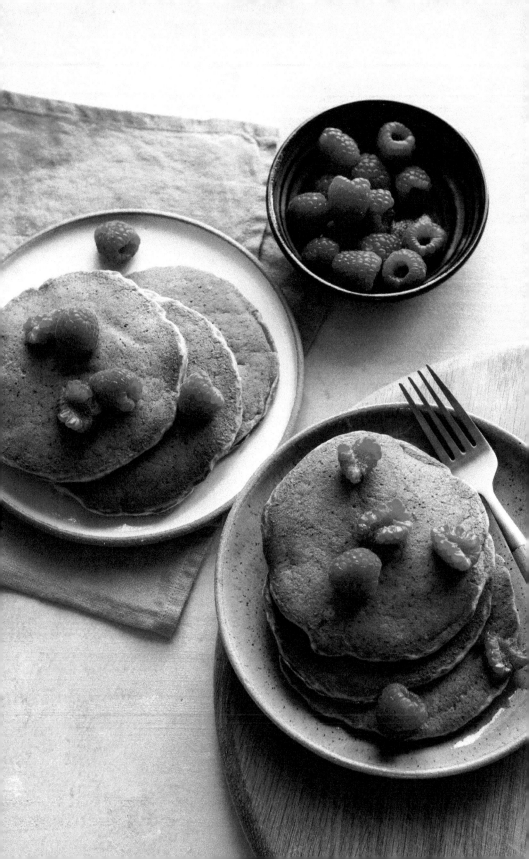

Chapter 4

Breakfast

Butternut Squash Nest Eggs

Serves 2 / Prep time: 5 mins / Cook time: 10 mins

DAIRY-FREE   GLUTEN-FREE   NUT-FREE   SOY-FREE

HYPOGLYCEMIA POWER FOOD, INSOMNIA, LOW-FODMAP FOR IBS, BRAIN FOG, MOOD BOOSTER, HASHIMOTO'S POWER FOOD, FIBROMYALGIA POWER FOOD, TOXIN BUSTER

This breakfast always ends up on my busy clients' menus. You can purchase spiralized butternut squash (or zucchini) to save time in the morning. Although this is on the breakfast menu, it's also great for lunch and dinner. The most important part of making this recipe is to cover the pan with the lid to steam the butternut squash and eggs. Feel free to add Quick Pickled Red Onions (page 150), Peruvian Green Spicy Sauce (page 147), or both.

½ tablespoon extra-virgin olive oil
1 garlic clove, minced ◆ / ■
1 cup spiralized butternut
   squash ◆ / ■

Kosher salt
Freshly ground black pepper
2 large eggs
1 cup baby arugula, for serving

1. Heat the olive oil in a large skillet over medium-low heat.

2. Add the garlic and sauté for 1 to 2 minutes, then add the spiralized butternut squash in 2 piles to form "nests."

3. Season with salt and pepper.

4. Crack an egg into each nest, cover the skillet with a lid, and cook for about 5 minutes, or until the squash is soft.

5. Serve warm over a bed of arugula.

Substitution Tip: If you have IBS or Fibromyalgia, omit the garlic (if desired, use garlic-infused olive oil instead of regular olive oil). Replace the spiralized butternut squash with spiralized zucchini.

Per serving: Calories: 129; Total fat: 8g; Carbohydrates: 9g; Fiber: 2g; Protein: 7g; Calcium: 77mg; Vitamin D: 36mcg; Vitamin B12: 0mcg; Iron: 1mg; Zinc: 1mg

Apple-Chia Power Muffins

Makes 12 muffins / **Prep time: 15 mins** / **Cook time: 25 mins**

DAIRY-FREE   GLUTEN-FREE   SOY-FREE

HYPOGLYCEMIA POWER FOOD, INSOMNIA, LOW-FODMAP FOR IBS, BRAIN
FOG, MOOD BOOSTER, HASHIMOTO'S POWER FOOD, FIBROMYALGIA
POWER FOOD, TOXIN BUSTER

This is my go-to breakfast or snack whenever my schedule is hectic. This
recipe makes 12 muffins (or 48 mini muffins). To reheat, microwave these
muffins for 30 seconds each. Pair them with Red Berry Jam (page 152) for a
bit more sweetness, or enjoy with a cup of fresh berries for extra fiber.

Olive oil or coconut oil, for greasing
  the muffin tin
2½ cups almond flour ◆
1 cup gluten-free oat flour (or
  pulverized gluten-free rolled oats)
½ cup walnuts
¼ cup chia seeds, plus 2 tablespoons
2 teaspoons ground cinnamon

1 teaspoon baking soda
¼ teaspoon kosher salt
3 large eggs
2 cups grated Fuji apples (2 or
  3 apples) ◆
1 cup mashed bananas (about
  1½ bananas)
6 tablespoons extra-virgin olive oil

1. Preheat the oven to 350°F. Line a 12-cup muffin tin with muffin liners or
   grease each cup with coconut or olive oil.

2. In a large mixing bowl, combine the almond flour, oat flour, walnuts,
   ¼ cup of chia seeds, cinnamon, baking soda, and salt.

3. In a separate medium mixing bowl, combine the eggs, grated apples,
   mashed bananas, and olive oil.

4. Add the wet ingredients to the dry ingredients and mix until
   just incorporated.

5. Spoon the batter into each muffin cup, filling them to the brim. Sprinkle
   the tops with the remaining 2 tablespoons of chia seeds.

6. Bake for 25 minutes (or 15 minutes for mini muffins), or until the tops are
   just golden brown and a tester inserted into the center comes out clean.

continued ››

7. Serve the muffins warm, and cool leftovers completely before storing. Store leftover muffins in an airtight container or resealable bag. Refrigerate them for up to 1 week or freeze them for 2 to 3 months.

Prep Tip: If you have rolled oats at home, you can use a food processor or blender to pulverize them into a coarse oat flour.

Substitution Tip: If you have IBS, replace the almond flour with more oat flour, and replace the apples with carrots.

Per serving (1 muffin): Calories: 281; Total fat: 20g; Carbohydrates: 21g; Fiber: 6g; Protein: 7g; Calcium: 100mg; Vitamin D: 9mcg; Vitamin B12: 0mcg; Iron: 2mg; Zinc: 1mg

Connor's "Cereal" Granola

Makes 8 cups (24 servings) / **Prep time: 10 mins** / **Cook time: 25 mins**

DAIRY-FREE   GLUTEN-FREE   SOY-FREE

HYPOGLYCEMIA POWER FOOD, INSOMNIA, BRAIN FOG, LOW-FODMAP
FOR IBS, MOOD BOOSTER

When you are following a very specific diet, traveling can be a challenge—but being prepared can help. I encourage my clients to carry snacks with them wherever they go. This big-batch granola is my son Connor's favorite snack to travel with. It's so versatile: You can add it to smoothies, enjoy it with plant-based milk and berries like cereal, or eat it straight out of the bag.

4 cups gluten-free rolled oats
1 cup chopped pecans
½ cup pepitas
½ teaspoon ground cinnamon
¼ cup chia seeds
¼ cup pure maple syrup
¼ cup melted coconut oil or
  extra-virgin olive oil

1 teaspoon alcohol- and sugar-free
  vanilla extract
½ cup Creamy Vanilla Cashew Milk
  (page 148), for serving
½ cup fresh berries of your choice,
  for serving

1. Preheat the oven to 350°F and line 2 large rimmed baking sheets with parchment paper.

2. In a large mixing bowl, combine the oats, pecans, pepitas, cinnamon, chia seeds, maple syrup, oil, and vanilla and stir to mix well.

3. Spread the mixture in an even layer onto both baking sheets and bake for 25 minutes, stirring halfway through.

4. Cool the granola completely before storing or serving. To serve, put ⅓ cup of the granola in a small bowl and add ½ cup of Creamy Vanilla Cashew Milk and ½ cup of fresh berries.

5. Store for up to a month in airtight glass jars or resealable bags in a dry, cool place.

Per serving: Calories: 187; Total fat: 9g; Carbohydrates: 21g; Fiber: 4g; Protein: 6g; Calcium: 37mg; Vitamin D: 0mcg; Vitamin B12: 0mcg; Iron: 2mg; Zinc: 2mg

Fluffiest Raspberry Pancakes

Serves 4 / **Prep time: 5 mins** / **Cook time: 15 mins**

DAIRY-FREE   GLUTEN-FREE   NUT-FREE   SOY-FREE

HYPOGLYCEMIA POWER FOOD, INSOMNIA, BRAIN FOG, LOW-FODMAP
FOR IBS, MOOD BOOSTER, HASHIMOTO'S POWER FOOD, FIBROMYALGIA
POWER FOOD, TOXIN BUSTER

Traditional store-bought pancake mix often contains a large amount of sugar
in addition to refined grains and chemicals that can cause inflammation.
If making pancakes from scratch feels like a lot of work, make the batter
ahead and store it in the refrigerator for up to 3 days. These pancakes are
slightly crispy on the outside and fluffy on the inside—they pair perfectly
with nut butter and Red Berry Jam (page 152).

¾ cup unsweetened oat milk or other
plant-based milk

2 tablespoons apple cider vinegar

1 cup buckwheat flour

1 teaspoon aluminum-free
baking powder

½ teaspoon baking soda

⅛ teaspoon kosher salt

1 large egg

2 tablespoons coconut oil, plus more
for cooking

1½ cups frozen raspberries

2 tablespoons pure maple syrup (skip
for Week 3, Week 4, and the Flare-Up
Meal Plan)

1. In a medium mixing bowl, combine the plant-based milk and apple cider
   vinegar to make "buttermilk." Stir and allow it to rest for 5 minutes, or
   until it curdles.

2. Add the buckwheat flour, baking powder, baking soda, salt, egg,
   2 tablespoons of coconut oil, the raspberries, and maple syrup (if using)
   to the buttermilk mixture and stir until just combined.

3. Heat a drizzle of coconut oil in a 10-inch nonstick pan over medium
   heat. Ladle ¼ cup of the batter into the pan for each pancake (or less for
   smaller pancakes). Cook the pancakes for 2 to 4 minutes, or until bub-
   bles form, then flip and cook for 2 minutes, or until golden brown on both
   sides. Serve immediately.

A Closer Look: When using plant-based milk for pancake batter, it's helpful to add a little bit of vinegar to create a plant-based buttermilk. This will make your pancakes nice and fluffy without using dairy.

Substitution Tip: The recipe calls for buckwheat flour, but sorghum or teff flour can be substituted as well. If you use oat flour, your pancakes might not hold together well, so combine it with other gluten-free flours. If you have IBS, use only 1 cup of raspberries.

Per serving: Calories: 258; Total fat: 10g; Carbohydrates: 39g; Fiber: 5g; Protein: 7g; Calcium: 99mg; Vitamin D: 9mcg; Vitamin B12: 0mcg; Iron: 2mg; Zinc: 1mg

Creamy Chocolate Oatmeal

Serves 2 / Prep time: 5 mins / Cook time: 10 mins

DAIRY-FREE   GLUTEN-FREE   SOY-FREE

HYPOGLYCEMIA POWER FOOD, INSOMNIA, BRAIN FOG, LOW-FODMAP
FOR IBS, MOOD BOOSTER, HASHIMOTO'S POWER FOOD, TOXIN BUSTER

Once, after a weekend of birthday celebrations and lots of chocolate cake,
my son asked whether we could make chocolate-flavored oatmeal for breakfast. We experimented and came up with this pretty amazing recipe. Hearty
oats and plant-based milk come together to make a creamy, rich breakfast.

½ cup gluten-free rolled oats
2 tablespoons chia seeds
1 cup plant-based milk
1 teaspoon unsweetened
   cocoa powder

1 tablespoon pure maple syrup
   (skip for Week 3, Week 4, and
   the Flare-Up Meal Plan)
1 teaspoon cashew butter ◆
1 tablespoon chopped walnuts,
   for serving
⅓ cup fresh berries, for serving

1. In a small saucepan, combine the oats, chia seeds, plant-based milk,
   cocoa powder, maple syrup (if using), and cashew butter. Place the
   saucepan over medium-high heat and stir frequently for 3 to 5 minutes,
   or until the mixture comes to a boil.

2. Once the mixture starts to bubble, reduce the heat to low and cook for
   3 to 5 minutes, stirring occasionally, or until the mixture becomes thick
   and creamy.

3. Serve the oatmeal warm, topped with the walnuts and berries. Refrigerate
   leftover oatmeal in an airtight container for up to 1 week and microwave
   for 1 to 2 minutes per serving to reheat.

Stretch Tip: This oatmeal recipe can be easily doubled or tripled to use as
breakfast all week.

Substitution Tip: If you have IBS, use peanut butter instead of
cashew butter.

Per serving: Calories: 369; Total fat: 13g; Carbohydrates: 51g; Fiber: 11g; Protein: 14g;
Calcium: 159mg; Vitamin D: 0mcg; Vitamin B12: 0mcg; Iron: 4mg; Zinc: 3mg

Uplift Green Smoothie

Serves 1 / **Prep time: 5 mins** / **Cook time: 5 mins**

DAIRY-FREE   GLUTEN-FREE   SOY-FREE

HYPOGLYCEMIA POWER FOOD, INSOMNIA, BRAIN FOG, LOW-FODMAP
FOR IBS, MOOD BOOSTER, FIBROMYALGIA POWER FOOD, TOXIN BUSTER

This green smoothie is perfect for mornings when you wake up craving something refreshing and uplifting. Pineapple is high in antioxidants that can boost your immune system and suppress inflammation, as well as a group of enzymes (called bromelain) that aid digestion. You can add the protein powder to make it more substantial, but if you want to enjoy it as a snack, feel free to omit it.

1 cup packed baby spinach
  (or ½ cup frozen spinach)
½ cup fresh or frozen
  pineapple chunks
½ tablespoon cashew butter ◆
1 tablespoon chia seeds

½ cup coconut water (or unsweetened
  plant-based milk, if adding
  protein powder)
½ scoop pea protein powder ◆
  (optional)
¼ cup water
¼ cup ice

1. Combine the spinach, pineapple, cashew butter, chia seeds, coconut water, pea protein powder (if using), and water in a blender. Blend on high until smooth.

2. Add the ice and blend until thick. Serve immediately.

Substitution Tip: If you have IBS, use peanut butter instead of cashew butter and omit the protein powder.

A Closer Look: Although pineapple is not high in fiber, its nutrient components are perfect for addressing adrenal fatigue symptoms. Try replacing pineapple with another fruit, or add frozen cauliflower for extra fiber and nutrients.

Per serving: Calories: 267; Total fat: 10g; Carbohydrates: 31g; Fiber: 10g; Protein: 18g; Calcium: 204mg; Vitamin D: 0mcg; Vitamin B12: 0mcg; Iron: 6mg; Zinc: 3mg

Muffin Tin Frittatas

Serves 4 (makes 12 egg muffins) / **Prep time: 10 mins**
Cook time: 20 mins

DAIRY-FREE   GLUTEN-FREE   NUT-FREE   SOY-FREE

INSOMNIA, MOOD BOOSTER, BRAIN FOG, TOXIN BUSTER

Many of my clients have told me they buy single-serving egg cups, wraps, or hard-boiled eggs at convenience stores because they don't have time to make breakfast. This recipe was designed with those clients in mind. You can make these ahead and microwave them for 1 to 2 minutes to reheat—though they're also good cold! They make great breakfasts on the go.

Olive oil or coconut oil, for greasing the muffin tin

8 large eggs, beaten

⅛ teaspoon kosher salt

⅛ teaspoon freshly ground black pepper

2 cups baby spinach, chopped

1 cup halved cherry tomatoes ●

1 small to medium shallot, finely chopped ◆ / ■

1 bell pepper, seeded and chopped ●

1. Preheat the oven to 350°F. Line a 12-cup muffin tin with muffin liners or grease each cup with olive oil.

2. In a medium mixing bowl, combine the eggs, salt, and pepper and beat until slightly foamy and liquefied.

3. Divide the spinach, tomatoes, shallot, and bell pepper evenly among the muffin cups. Pour the eggs over the vegetables in each muffin cup, filling them almost to the top.

4. Bake for 20 minutes, or until the frittata muffins are set.

5. Serve immediately or refrigerate leftover frittata muffins in an airtight container for up to 4 days.

Stretch Tip: You can use any leftover fresh or cooked vegetables as a filling for this recipe. If the vegetables look soggy or droopy, sauté them for 3 to 4 minutes to crisp them up before you add them to the muffin cups.

Substitution Tip: If you have IBS or Fibromyalgia, replace the shallot with the green portion of 1 scallion. If you have Hashimoto's, omit the cherry tomatoes and bell pepper or replace them with diced zucchini.

Per serving: Calories: 170; Total fat: 10g; Carbohydrates: 6g; Fiber: 1g; Protein: 14g; Calcium: 81mg; Vitamin D: 82mcg; Vitamin B12: 1mcg; Iron: 3mg; Zinc: 2mg

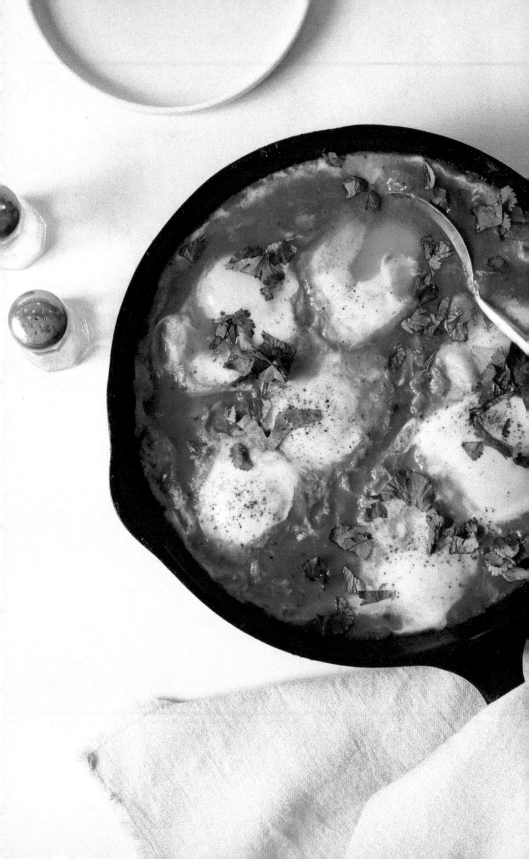

Chapter 5

Lunch

Shakshuka

Serves 2 / Prep time: 5 mins / Cook time: 20 mins

DAIRY-FREE   GLUTEN-FREE   NUT-FREE   SOY-FREE

HYPOGLYCEMIA POWER FOOD, INSOMNIA, BRAIN FOG, MOOD BOOSTER, LOW-FODMAP FOR IBS, FIBROMYALGIA POWER FOOD, TOXIN BUSTER

This flexible dish is a quick go-to lunch, breakfast, or dinner and can be easily scaled up to feed a larger group. The chickpeas provide fiber and carbohydrates for sustained energy. Feel free to add any vegetable you have on hand, like zucchini, spinach, mushrooms, or asparagus.

1 tablespoon extra-virgin olive oil
2 tablespoons minced garlic ◆ / ■
1 teaspoon ground cumin
½ cup diced bell peppers
¼ teaspoon kosher salt

2 cups (16 ounces) canned unsalted diced tomatoes
½ cup canned unsalted chickpeas, rinsed and drained
4 large eggs
2 tablespoons chopped fresh parsley

1. Heat the olive oil in a large skillet over medium-high heat. Add the garlic, cumin, bell peppers, and salt and sauté for about 5 minutes, or until the peppers are softened.

2. Add the tomatoes (with their juices) and chickpeas and cook for 10 minutes, stirring occasionally.

3. Make 4 small wells in the sauce and crack an egg into each well.

4. Cover the skillet with a lid and cook for 5 minutes, or until the egg whites are opaque. Remove the skillet from the heat and garnish with the chopped parsley. Serve immediately.

Too Tired to Cook: To speed this recipe up, use premade tomato sauce or Roasted Eggplant Ragù (page 119) instead of canned tomatoes and skip the other vegetables. Add the sauce to the skillet with olive oil, warm it, and just add eggs!

Substitution Tip: If you have IBS or Fibromyalgia, omit the garlic and use garlic-infused olive oil.

Per serving: Calories: 321; Total fat: 17g; Carbohydrates: 26g; Fiber: 9g; Protein: 18g; Calcium: 182mg; Vitamin D: 72mcg; Vitamin B12: 1mcg; Iron: 5mg; Zinc: 2mg

Lentil-Spinach Fritters

Serves 4 / Prep time: 10 mins, plus 1 hour soaking / Cook time: 15 mins

DAIRY-FREE   GLUTEN-FREE   NUT-FREE   SOY-FREE

HYPOGLYCEMIA POWER FOOD, INSOMNIA, BRAIN FOG, MOOD BOOSTER, LOW-FODMAP FOR IBS, HASHIMOTO'S POWER FOOD, FIBROMYALGIA POWER FOOD, TOXIN BUSTER

I encourage all my clients to incorporate a variety of plant-based proteins into their diets. I love lentils for this purpose, because they provide protein as well as fiber, which is essential for good gut health. These crispy-on-the-outside, soft-on-the-inside fritters are a favorite in my family—they never make it to a plate, because we all stand around the stove and eat them straight out of the pan!

1 cup red lentils, soaked in warm water for at least 1 hour and then drained
½ red onion, diced ◆ / ▧
½ teaspoon ground cumin
½ teaspoon ground coriander
½ teaspoon minced fresh ginger

½ cup finely chopped spinach
¼ cup chopped fresh cilantro
⅛ teaspoon kosher salt
⅛ teaspoon freshly ground black pepper
Extra-virgin olive oil, for frying

1. In a food processor, pulse the lentils until a coarse mixture forms.

2. In a small bowl, combine the lentils, red onion, cumin, coriander, ginger, spinach, cilantro, salt, and pepper. Mix well.

3. Heat a drizzle of olive oil in a large skillet over medium heat. Drop 2 tablespoons of the lentil mixture per fritter into the skillet to loosely form bite-size fritters. Cook the fritters for about 3 minutes on each side, or until golden brown all over. Serve immediately.

Prep Tip: Premake the fritter mixture ahead and keep it refrigerated for up to 3 days to make fresh fritters as desired. Reheat already-cooked fritters in a skillet to warm them through.

Substitution Tip: If you have IBS or Fibromyalgia, replace the red onion with the green portion of 1 or 2 scallions.

Per serving: Calories: 244; Total fat: 8g; Carbohydrates: 33g; Fiber: 6g; Protein: 12g; Calcium: 55mg; Vitamin D: 0mcg; Vitamin B12: 0mcg; Iron: 4mg; Zinc: 2mg

Quinoa and Arugula Salad with Vegetables

Serves 6 / Prep time: 10 mins, plus quinoa cooking time

DAIRY-FREE   GLUTEN-FREE   SOY-FREE

HYPOGLYCEMIA POWER FOOD, INSOMNIA, BRAIN FOG, LOW-FODMAP FOR IBS, MOOD BOOSTER, HASHIMOTO'S POWER FOOD, FIBROMYALGIA POWER FOOD, TOXIN BUSTER

Quinoa is considered a "complete" protein because it contains all the essential amino acids (just like animal-source protein). I love making this salad over the summer with peak-season tomatoes that are ripe, sweet, and super juicy. When you make this salad in the summer, skip the vinaigrette, and use olive oil, salt, and pepper. This salad pairs perfectly with a hard-boiled or fried egg for even more protein.

2 cups cooked quinoa
2 cups fresh baby arugula
1 cup halved cherry tomatoes ●
1 cup chopped seedless cucumber
1 small to medium shallot, finely chopped ◆ / ■

1 cup canned unsalted chickpeas, rinsed and drained
¼ cup pine nuts
¼ cup Dijon Mustard Vinaigrette (page 151)

In a bowl, combine the quinoa, arugula, cherry tomatoes, cucumber, shallot, chickpeas, pine nuts, and vinaigrette. Toss to combine. Refrigerate leftovers for up to 3 days.

Prep Tip: Make the quinoa in advance so you can put this salad together in less than 10 minutes. Store cooked grains in your freezer or refrigerator to significantly cut down on cooking time. Cooked grains can last 3 to 4 days in your refrigerator.

Substitution Tip: If you have IBS or Fibromyalgia, replace the shallot with the green portion of 1 scallion. If you have Hashimoto's, omit the cherry tomatoes.

Per serving: Calories: 232; Total fat: 15g; Carbohydrates: 23g; Fiber: 5g; Protein: 6g; Calcium: 41mg; Vitamin D: 0mcg; Vitamin B12: 0mcg; Iron: 2mg; Zinc: 2mg

One-Pot Chicken and Quinoa

Serves 6 / Prep time: 10 mins / Cook time: 30 mins

DAIRY-FREE GLUTEN-FREE NUT-FREE SOY-FREE

HYPOGLYCEMIA POWER FOOD, INSOMNIA, BRAIN FOG, MOOD BOOSTER, TOXIN BUSTER

A true oldie but goodie, this chicken and quinoa recipe is one I have been making for years. Don't let the 30-minute cooking time fool you—this easy one-pot meal practically cooks itself. The chicken comes out soft and tender—even my toddler loves it! I recommend an Instant Pot (or other pressure cooker) for this dish, but if you don't have one, I've included instructions for stovetop cooking in the Prep Tip after the recipe.

1 tablespoon extra-virgin olive oil
3 garlic cloves, minced ◆ / ▓
1 cup chopped shallots ◆ / ▓
1 tablespoon ground cumin
1 tablespoon ground coriander
1 pound boneless, skinless chicken thighs, diced
1 (15-ounce) can unsalted black beans (or kidney beans), rinsed and drained

1 cup uncooked quinoa
1 medium zucchini, finely diced
1⅓ cups unsalted chicken broth (or 3 cups if cooking on the stovetop)
1½ cups tomato sauce ●
1 cup fresh cilantro, coarsely chopped, for garnish

1. Turn on your pressure cooker and press the Sauté setting (or see the stovetop instructions in the Prep Tip). Combine the oil, garlic, and shallots and sauté for about 3 minutes, or until the shallots are translucent.

2. Add the cumin, coriander, chicken, beans, quinoa, zucchini, chicken broth, and tomato sauce. Stir to ensure that all ingredients are submerged in the broth.

3. Close the lid and press the Poultry setting (high pressure), or see the stovetop instructions. Allow the pressure cooker to pressurize (about 10 minutes) and cook (about 15 minutes).

4. Serve hot, garnished with the cilantro. Refrigerate leftovers for up to 1 week.

continued ››

Prep Tip: If you don't have an Instant Pot, use a large pot, and cook on the stovetop over medium heat. Follow the same instructions, but be sure to adjust the amount of broth to account for evaporation and to ensure that the quinoa and chicken can cook. After step 2, allow the broth to boil, reduce the heat to low, cover, and cook for about 30 minutes, or until the liquid is mostly evaporated and the chicken and quinoa are cooked through.

Substitution Tip: If you have IBS or Fibromyalgia, replace the garlic and shallots with the green portion of 1 or 2 scallions. If you have Hashimoto's, replace the tomato sauce with an additional 1½ cups of chicken broth.

Per serving: Calories: 316; Total fat: 8g; Carbohydrates: 38g; Fiber: 8g; Protein: 25g; Calcium: 66mg; Vitamin D: 1mcg; Vitamin B12: 1mcg; Iron: 5mg; Zinc: 3mg

Crunchy Summer Salad

Serves 4 / Prep time: 15 mins

DAIRY-FREE   GLUTEN-FREE   SOY-FREE

HYPOGLYCEMIA POWER FOOD, INSOMNIA, BRAIN FOG, MOOD BOOSTER, HASHIMOTO'S POWER FOOD, TOXIN BUSTER

Fresh, crunchy vegetables are all I want to eat when it's warm outside. I don't usually recommend plain leafy green salads to my clients—I actually discourage it. Greens lack fiber, fat, and protein, and you'll be hungry again an hour after eating them. Instead, I recommend a salad with a variety of non-starchy vegetables and healthy fats and protein (like avocado and nuts) to keep you satiated and your energy level up.

8 asparagus spears, woody ends peeled or removed, cut into bite-size lengths

1 cup green beans, trimmed and halved (about 25 beans)

2 cups baby spinach

6 radishes, thinly sliced

1 red bell pepper, halved, stemmed, and seeded ●

1 cup sliced seedless cucumber

⅛ cup pine nuts (or other nuts or seeds of your choice)

¼ cup Dijon Mustard Vinaigrette (page 151)

1 avocado, pitted and sliced

1. In a medium bowl, combine the asparagus spears, green beans, baby spinach, radishes, bell pepper, cucumber, and pine nuts.

2. If serving immediately, toss with the vinaigrette and top with the sliced avocado. If serving later, follow the storage instructions in the Prep Tip.

Prep Tip: This salad can be put together in a large storage container. If you premake this salad, add the avocado and dressing only when you're ready to eat it. This salad is perfect on its own or with a simple protein such as chicken, tofu, beans, or fish.

Substitution Tip: If you have Hashimoto's, omit the bell pepper.

Per serving: Calories: 207; Total fat: 19g; Carbohydrates: 12g; Fiber: 7g; Protein: 4g; Calcium: 41mg; Vitamin D: 0mcg; Vitamin B12: 0mcg; Iron: 1mg; Zinc: 1mg

Hearty Black Bean Burgers

Serves 4 / Prep time: 15 mins / Cook time: 15 mins

DAIRY-FREE   GLUTEN-FREE   NUT-FREE   SOY-FREE

HYPOGLYCEMIA POWER FOOD, INSOMNIA, MOOD BOOSTER, HASHIMOTO'S POWER FOOD, TOXIN BUSTER

I originally created this recipe for my son, but it quickly became a family favorite. To save time, I use a mini food processor to do all the chopping prep work. You can serve these burgers on gluten-free bread, in lettuce wraps, or even on a salad. Try making mini burgers to serve as sliders with butter lettuce and sliced tomatoes. For a spicy kick, drizzle cooked patties with Peruvian Green Spicy Sauce (see page 147).

1 (15-ounce) can black beans, rinsed and drained

½ cup cooked brown rice or quinoa

½ red bell pepper, diced ●

1 small to medium shallot, finely chopped ◆ / ■

1 garlic clove, minced ◆ / ■

2 large eggs

1 teaspoon ground cumin

¼ teaspoon kosher salt

¼ cup fresh parsley, finely chopped

¼ cup fresh cilantro, finely chopped

1 scallion, green and white parts, thinly sliced

⅓ cup gluten-free bread crumbs, such as chickpea

Extra-virgin olive oil, for frying

1. Dry the rinsed and drained black beans on a paper towel.

2. In a food processor, combine the beans, rice, bell pepper, shallot, and garlic and pulse until finely chopped.

3. Add the eggs, cumin, salt, parsley, cilantro, scallion, and gluten-free bread crumbs. Pulse until a well-combined dough forms. Form the mixture into 4 palm-size patties.

4. Drizzle olive oil in a skillet over medium heat. Fry the patties for about 3 minutes on each side, or until the exterior is browned and crispy. Serve warm or let cool before storing.

Prep Tip: These patties can be premade and frozen, uncooked, for up to 2 months (thaw them as needed before frying). If you don't have a food processor, use a blender on the Pulse setting and stir or shake frequently to avoid puréeing the ingredients.

Substitution Tip: If you have Hashimoto's, omit the bell pepper. If you have IBS or Fibromyalgia, replace the garlic and shallot with the green portion of 1 or 2 additional scallions. If you can't find chickpea or gluten-free bread crumbs, increase the cooked brown rice to ⅔ cup.

Per serving: Calories: 200; Total fat: 5g; Carbohydrates: 27g; Fiber: 7g; Protein: 11g; Calcium: 53mg; Vitamin D: 18mcg; Vitamin B12: 0mcg; Iron: 3mg; Zinc: 1mg

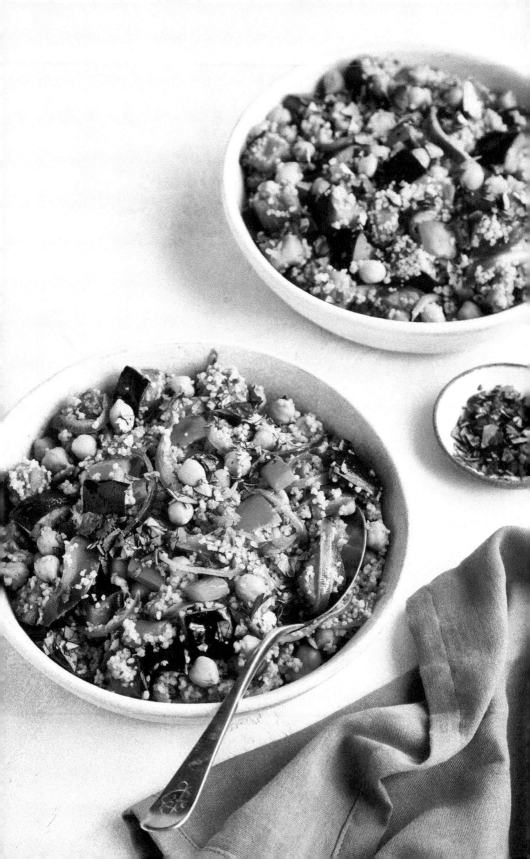

Chapter 6

Hearty Bowls

Roasted Vegetable Grain Bowl

Serves 2 / **Prep time: 5 mins** / **Cook time: 20 mins**

DAIRY-FREE   GLUTEN-FREE   NUT-FREE   SOY-FREE

HYPOGLYCEMIA POWER FOOD, INSOMNIA, BRAIN FOG, MOOD BOOSTER, HASHIMOTO'S POWER FOOD, TOXIN BUSTER

I grew up eating grain bowls with vegetables, so this recipe feels like home. As a dietitian today, I recommend dishes like this one to my clients because they are nutritionally balanced and simple to prepare. You can use leftovers or any vegetables you have around in this recipe, like butternut squash, zucchini, asparagus, or onions. This bowl (and any grain bowl) is great drizzled with sauce—try the Peruvian Green Spicy Sauce (page 147).

1 cup mixed vegetables of your choice, cut into 1-inch dice

3 tablespoons extra-virgin olive oil, divided

2 large eggs

1 cup cooked quinoa (about ⅓ cup uncooked), for serving

½ avocado, pitted and thinly sliced

4 radishes, thinly sliced

2 cups baby spinach

½ cup Quick Pickled Red Onions (page 150) ◆ / ▣

1. Preheat the oven to 400°F and line a large rimmed baking sheet with parchment paper.

2. In a mixing bowl, toss the diced vegetables with 1 tablespoon of olive oil. Spread into a single layer on the prepared baking sheet and bake for 20 minutes, or until golden brown.

3. Heat the remaining 2 tablespoons of olive oil in a nonstick skillet over medium heat. Fry the eggs to your liking (I prefer over-easy) and set them aside.

4. Divide the quinoa between 2 large serving bowls and top with the roasted vegetables, avocado, radishes, baby spinach, fried eggs, and pickled red onions. Serve warm or cold.

Prep Tip: This recipe can be made with any vegetables and grains you have, so use this dish to revitalize your leftovers to make a delicious lunch or dinner.

Substitution Tip: If you have IBS or Fibromyalgia, skip the Quick Pickled Red Onions—if desired, add the green portions of 1 or 2 scallions, finely chopped.

Per serving: Calories: 512; Total fat: 34g; Carbohydrates: 39g; Fiber: 12g; Protein: 15g; Calcium: 103mg; Vitamin D: 36mcg; Vitamin B12: 0mcg; Iron: 4mg; Zinc: 3mg

Creamy Masoor Dal Grain Bowl

Serves 4 to 6 / **Prep time: 5 mins** / **Cook time: 20 mins**

DAIRY-FREE   GLUTEN-FREE   NUT-FREE   SOY-FREE

HYPOGLYCEMIA POWER FOOD, INSOMNIA, BRAIN FOG, MOOD BOOSTER, HASHIMOTO'S POWER FOOD, TOXIN BUSTER

When it comes to adrenal health, high-quality protein and fiber are crucial. Although red lentils (*masoor dal*) on their own are not a complete protein, they're even more nutritious than animal-sourced protein when served with whole grains. Dried split red lentils are convenient for this quick, rich grain bowl because they cook faster than many other dried beans.

2 tablespoons extra-virgin olive oil
1 tablespoon cumin seeds
½ red onion, chopped ◆ / ■
1 tablespoon ground coriander
1½ teaspoons ground turmeric
2 tablespoons minced garlic ◆ / ■
1 tablespoon minced fresh ginger
2 cups dried red lentils
4 cups unsalted vegetable broth

4 cups water
Salt
Freshly ground black pepper
2 to 3 cups cooked whole grains of
   your choice, such as brown rice
   or quinoa
½ cup chopped fresh cilantro,
   for garnish

1. Heat the olive oil in a large pot over medium-high heat. Once the oil is hot, add the cumin seeds and fry for about 30 seconds, or just until fragrant.

2. Add the red onion and sauté for about 2 minutes, or until the onion is beginning to brown. Add the coriander, turmeric, garlic, and ginger and sauté for about 1 minute, or until fragrant.

3. Add the lentils, broth, and water. Cook, stirring occasionally, for about 15 minutes, or until the lentils are creamy. Add salt and pepper to taste.

4. To assemble the bowls, combine ½ cup of brown rice or quinoa and ½ cup of the dal in each bowl and garnish with the cilantro.

Prep Tip: This is a great recipe to prepare in advance of a busy week. You can make the lentils and grains ahead of time and refrigerate both separately for up to 4 days. Reheat individual servings as necessary.

Substitution Tip: If you don't have cumin seeds, add the same amount of ground cumin along with the other spices in step 2. If you have IBS or Fibromyalgia, replace the garlic and onion with the green portions of 3 or 4 scallions.

Per serving: Calories: 547; Total fat: 10g; Carbohydrates: 90g; Fiber: 13g; Protein: 26g; Calcium: 84mg; Vitamin D: 0mcg; Vitamin B12: 0mcg; Iron: 9mg; Zinc: 4mg

Chicken Tikka Masala Grain Bowl

Serves 8 / **Prep time: 10 mins** / **Cook time: 20 mins**

DAIRY-FREE   GLUTEN-FREE   NUT-FREE   SOY-FREE

HYPOGLYCEMIA POWER FOOD, INSOMNIA, MOOD BOOSTER, BRAIN FOG, TOXIN BUSTER

Chicken tikka masala is a well-known Indian dish with a creamy tomato sauce base, often heavy in cream, butter, and dairy yogurt and usually served with white rice. For this healthier bowl, we'll use whole grains and replace the dairy with coconut yogurt. This is a great recipe to make ahead and enjoy all week.

1 tablespoon coconut oil

3 garlic cloves, minced ◆ / ▪

1 tablespoon grated fresh ginger

½ medium onion, diced ◆ / ▪

3 tablespoons tomato paste

1½ teaspoons garam masala

1½ teaspoons ground turmeric

1 cup unsalted chicken broth (or 2 cups if cooking on the stovetop)

1½ pounds boneless, skinless chicken breasts, diced

1 (15-ounce) can tomato sauce

½ cup plain coconut yogurt (no sugar or additives)

4 cups cooked whole grains of your choice, such as brown rice or quinoa

½ cup fresh cilantro, chopped, for garnish

1. Turn on your pressure cooker and press the Sauté setting (or see the stovetop instructions in the Prep Tip). Combine the coconut oil, garlic, ginger, and onion and sauté for 3 minutes, or until the onion is translucent.

2. Add the tomato paste, garam masala, and turmeric and cook for 1 more minute, or until fragrant.

3. Add the broth, chicken, tomato sauce, and yogurt and stir to combine.

4. Close the lid and press the Poultry setting (high pressure) or see the stovetop instructions. Allow the pressure cooker to pressurize and cook for 15 minutes.

5. To assemble the bowls, ladle the chicken tikka masala over ½ cup of your favorite grains per bowl and garnish with the cilantro. Refrigerate the chicken tikka masala and grains separately for up to 4 days.

Prep Tip: If you don't have an Instant Pot, use a large pot and cook on the stovetop over medium heat. Follow the same instructions, but in step 3, adjust the amount of broth to ensure that the chicken can cook through. After step 3, allow the mixture to almost reach a boil, then reduce the heat to low, cover, and simmer for 20 to 30 minutes, or until the chicken is cooked through and the sauce is creamy.

Substitution Tip: If you have IBS or Fibromyalgia, replace the garlic and onion with the green portions of 2 or 3 scallions.

Per serving: Calories: 251; Total fat: 5g; Carbohydrates: 27g; Fiber: 3g; Protein: 23g; Calcium: 47mg; Vitamin D: 1mcg; Vitamin B12: 0mcg; Iron: 2mg; Zinc: 1mg

Roasted Vegetable Fried Rice

Serves 6 / **Prep time: 5 mins** / **Cook time: 15 mins**

DAIRY-FREE   GLUTEN-FREE   NUT-FREE   SOY-FREE

HYPOGLYCEMIA POWER FOOD, INSOMNIA, MOOD BOOSTER,
HASHIMOTO'S POWER FOOD, TOXIN BUSTER

You can't go wrong with fried rice. Kids love it, it travels well, and it couldn't be easier to throw together. I love making fried rice to use up leftover roasted vegetables (like zucchini, string beans, asparagus, or carrots), but you don't need to add a lot of ingredients to make it super tasty. Even if your refrigerator is practically empty, you can make a super simple version of this recipe with just brown rice, eggs, scallions, and toasted sesame oil.

2 tablespoons olive oil

½ medium onion, chopped ◆ / ▣

2 garlic cloves, minced ◆ / ▣

½ tablespoon minced fresh ginger

2 to 4 cups leftover roasted vegetables of your choice, diced (or see the Substitution Tip)

2 tablespoons coconut aminos

2 large eggs, beaten

4 cups cooked whole grains of your choice, such as brown rice or quinoa

2 tablespoons toasted sesame oil

1. Heat the olive oil in a large skillet over medium heat. Add the onion, garlic, and ginger and sauté for about 3 minutes, or until the onion is translucent.

2. Add the vegetables and coconut aminos and cook for about 5 minutes, or until the vegetables are cooked through and beginning to soften.

3. Make a well in the middle of the mixture. Pour the eggs into the well and stir quickly to scramble, about 1 minute.

4. Once the eggs are almost cooked, stir them into the rest of the mixture to incorporate. Add the cooked grains and cook for 2 minutes, stirring frequently to warm through.

5. Turn off the heat, drizzle the rice with the sesame oil, and stir to combine. Serve warm in bowls.

Substitution Tip: If you don't have leftover vegetables on hand, use 5 asparagus spears, chopped and woody stems snapped off, and 1 medium zucchini, diced. If you have IBS or Fibromyalgia, replace the onion and garlic with the green portions of 3 or 4 scallions.

Prep Tip: This is my go-to menu item at the end of the week when I need to use up leftover cooked or fresh protein and produce. You can make this with any vegetables you have on hand—fresh, frozen, and leftover are all delicious.

Per serving: Calories: 274; Total fat: 12g; Carbohydrates: 36g; Fiber: 4g; Protein: 6g; Calcium: 38mg; Vitamin D: 12mcg; Vitamin B12: 0mcg; Iron: 1mg; Zinc: 1mg

Crispy Falafel Bowl

Serves 4 / **Prep time: 15 mins, plus soaking overnight** /
Cook time: 15 mins

DAIRY-FREE   GLUTEN-FREE   NUT-FREE   SOY-FREE

HYPOGLYCEMIA POWER FOOD, INSOMNIA, MOOD BOOSTER,
HASHIMOTO'S POWER FOOD, TOXIN BUSTER

My husband never tried falafel until he moved to New York City. Now that
we live here, he gets to eat it more than ever. The fresh herbs used in falafel
are a potent source of antioxidants that can protect cells, and falafel is so
versatile—it's served here in a hearty grain bowl, but it's also great in salads
and sandwiches. I prefer my falafel panfried, but it can also be baked at
425°F for 30 minutes.

1 cup dried red lentils or chickpeas,
   soaked and drained (see Prep Tip)
1 large shallot ◆ / ■
1 cup fresh parsley
3 garlic cloves ◆ / ■
1 teaspoon ground cumin
1 teaspoon kosher salt
½ teaspoon ground cardamom
¼ teaspoon freshly ground
   black pepper

2 teaspoons chickpea flour or other
   gluten-free flour
½ teaspoon baking soda
Extra-virgin olive oil, for frying
2 cups cooked whole grains of your
   choice, for serving
Creamy Tahini Dressing (page 146),
   for serving (optional)

1. Put the soaked and drained red lentils in a food processor or blender and
   pulse until they resemble a coarse meal. Transfer to a large bowl.

2. Put the shallot, parsley, and garlic in the same food processor and
   pulse until finely chopped. Add this mixture to the lentil mixture and stir
   to combine.

3. Add the cumin, salt, cardamom, pepper, flour, and baking soda and stir
   to incorporate.

4. Make falafel balls or patties, using 2 to 3 tablespoons of the mixture per
   ball. Roll the balls or patties gently with your hands, avoiding using too
   much pressure, so that they are fluffy.

5. Heat olive oil in a large skillet over medium heat. Fry the falafel for 2 to 3 minutes on each side, or until browned and crispy.

6. To assemble bowls, serve 2 or 3 falafel balls or patties over ½ cup of whole grains. Drizzle with the Creamy Tahini Dressing (if using).

Prep Tip: I have tried this recipe with lentils and chickpeas, and both work great. If using red lentils, soak them for about 1 hour. If using dried chickpeas, soak them overnight (8 to 12 hours). I don't recommend canned chickpeas for this recipe—they're too soft, and your falafel won't hold together.

Substitution Tip: If you have IBS or Fibromyalgia, replace the garlic and shallot with the green portions of 2 or 3 scallions.

Per serving: Calories: 358; Total fat: 9g; Carbohydrates: 56g; Fiber: 9g; Protein: 15g; Calcium: 65mg; Vitamin D: 0mcg; Vitamin B12: 0mcg; Iron: 5mg; Zinc: 3mg

Sautéed Mushroom and Quinoa Bowl

Serves 4 / Prep time: 5 mins / Cook time: less than 10 mins

DAIRY-FREE   GLUTEN-FREE   NUT-FREE   SOY-FREE

HYPOGLYCEMIA POWER FOOD, INSOMNIA, BRAIN FOG, MOOD BOOSTER, FIBROMYALGIA POWER FOOD, TOXIN BUSTER

I am a big fan of grain bowls—they're so easy to put together, and you can make them work with whatever leftover ingredients you have on hand. When I have leftovers to use up, this is my go-to recipe. The meaty texture of mushrooms fills out this dish. If you have IBS, you may be sensitive to some mushrooms, so read the Substitution Tip at the end of the recipe.

2 tablespoons extra-virgin olive oil

2 garlic cloves, minced ◆ / ■

½ cup finely chopped shallots ◆ / ■

2 portabella mushrooms, cleaned and cut into strips ◆

¼ cup sherry vinegar

1½ cups cooked quinoa (about ½ cup uncooked)

3 cups baby arugula

1. Heat the olive oil in a large skillet over medium-high heat.

2. Add the garlic and shallots and sauté for about 2 minutes, or until fragrant and slightly browned.

3. Add the mushrooms and vinegar and cook for 3 minutes, or until the mushrooms begin to get tender.

4. Add the cooked quinoa and arugula and sauté for 1 to 2 minutes, or just until the arugula is slightly wilted. Serve warm.

Substitution Tip: Sherry vinegar works best for this recipe, but you can also use balsamic vinegar. If you have IBS, replace the portabella mushrooms with oyster mushrooms. If you have IBS or Fibromyalgia, replace the shallots and garlic with the green portions of 3 or 4 scallions.

Per serving: Calories: 167; Total fat: 8g; Carbohydrates: 19g; Fiber: 3g; Protein: 4g; Calcium: 47mg; Vitamin D: 0mcg; Vitamin B12: 0mcg; Iron: 2mg; Zinc: 1mg

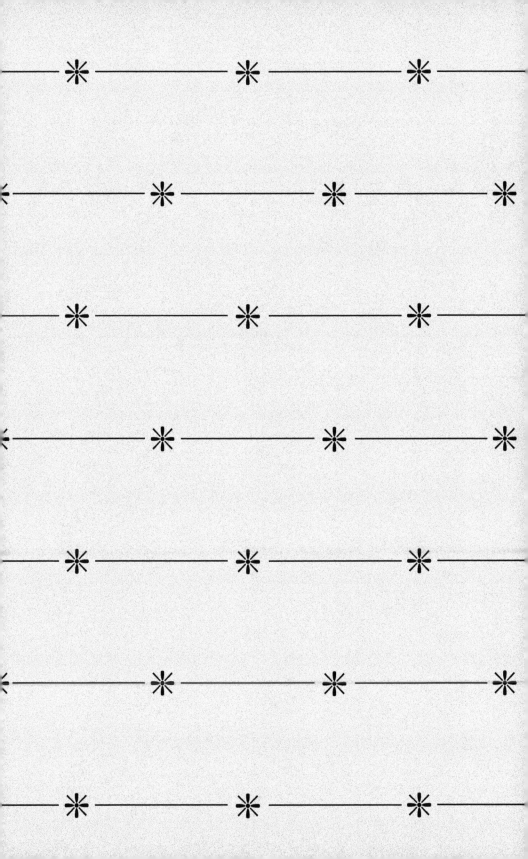

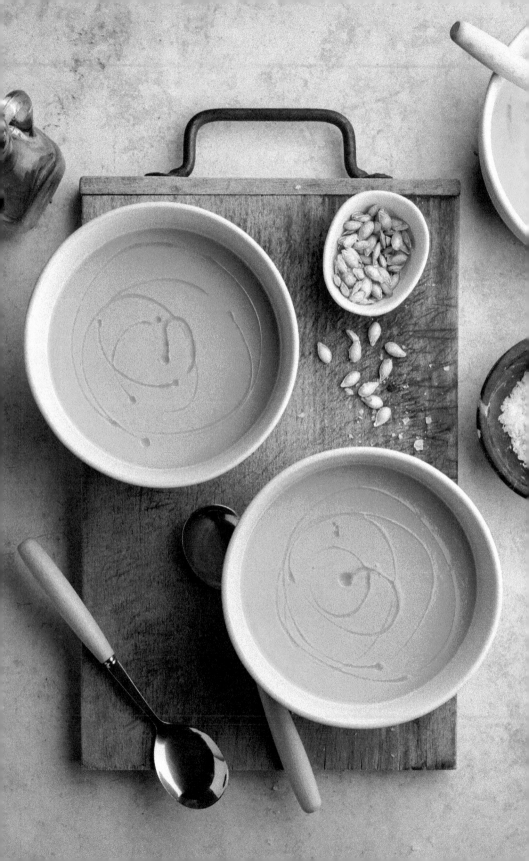

Chapter 7

Soups and Stews

Connor's Chicken Soup

Serves 8 / **Prep time: 10 mins** / **Cook time: 25 mins**

DAIRY-FREE   GLUTEN-FREE   NUT-FREE   SOY-FREE

HYPOGLYCEMIA POWER FOOD, INSOMNIA, MOOD BOOSTER, TOXIN BUSTER

As a busy mom, I consider one-pot meals my weeknight go-to. This recipe is quick to make and even quicker to clean up. Unlike typical chicken soup, this version uses lots of colorful vegetables that provide nutrients and fiber. I sometimes add ½ cup of uncooked quinoa or brown rice to make it heartier for my son. If you don't have an Instant Pot, use the stovetop instructions in the Prep Tip after the recipe.

1 pound boneless, skinless chicken thighs, diced or sliced
2 celery stalks, chopped
2 small to medium shallots, chopped ◆ / ■
1 medium tomato, diced ●
1 medium zucchini, diced
4 to 6 rainbow chard leaves, chopped
3 garlic cloves, chopped ◆ / ■

1 teaspoon grated fresh ginger
1 tablespoon ground cumin
1 tablespoon ground coriander
1 teaspoon ground turmeric
1 quart unsalted chicken stock
4 cups water
Kosher salt
Freshly ground black pepper

In the bowl of an Instant Pot or other pressure cooker, combine the chicken, celery, shallots, tomato, zucchini, rainbow chard, garlic, ginger, cumin, coriander, turmeric, chicken stock, and water. Close the lid, press the Poultry setting (high pressure), and allow the cooker to pressurize (about 10 minutes) and cook (about 15 minutes). Serve hot, sprinkled with salt and pepper to taste. Refrigerate leftovers for up to 4 days.

Prep Tip: If you don't have an Instant Pot, use a large pot on the stovetop. Drizzle in 1 tablespoon of olive oil and sauté the garlic, ginger, celery, and shallots for about 3 minutes over medium-high heat, or until the shallots are translucent. Cut the chicken into smaller pieces so it has time to cook through. Add the chicken and the rest of the ingredients to the pot and bring the soup to a boil; then cover, reduce the heat to low, and simmer for 20 minutes, or until the chicken is cooked through.

Substitution Tip: If you have IBS or Fibromyalgia, replace the shallots and garlic with the green portions of 2 or 3 scallions. If you have Hashimoto's, omit the tomato.

Per serving: Calories: 100; Total fat: 3g; Carbohydrates: 5g; Fiber: 1g; Protein: 13g; Calcium: 38mg; Vitamin D: 1mcg; Vitamin B12: 0mcg; Iron: 2mg; Zinc: 1mg

Chicken Bone Broth

Serves 8 (makes 2 quarts) / **Prep time: 10 mins** / **Cook time: 25 mins**

DAIRY-FREE   GLUTEN-FREE   NUT-FREE   SOY-FREE

INSOMNIA, MOOD BOOSTER, BRAIN FOG, HASHIMOTO'S POWER FOOD, TOXIN BUSTER

Bone broth is my go-to when I'm recovering from a cold or whenever I need to reset and recharge. The collagen peptides in bone broth serve as the building blocks of collagen and other proteins in the body. Store-bought bone broths can be really high in salt, and making your own is easy. I use an Instant Pot to save time, but you can also make this broth on the stovetop (see the Prep Tip after the recipe).

1 whole pasture-raised, organic heritage chicken, skin and giblets removed

2 celery stalks, cut into 4- to 5-inch sticks

1 head garlic, rinsed and cut in half ◆ / ■

1 thumb fresh ginger, cut into discs (about 1 tablespoon)

1 medium carrot, coarsely chopped

1 onion, quartered ◆ / ■

1 tablespoon whole black peppercorns

3 bay leaves

1. In an Instant Pot or other pressure cooker, combine the chicken, celery, garlic, ginger, carrot, onion, peppercorns, and bay leaves. Fill it with water to the 3-liter mark (about 3½ quarts), or until the chicken is covered. Press the Poultry setting (high pressure) and allow the pressure cooker to pressurize (about 10 minutes) and cook (about 15 minutes).

2. Once it is cooked, remove the chicken from the Instant Pot and separate the meat from the bones (it should fall off easily). Store the meat for another use. Reserve and store any vegetables you want to eat.

3. Strain the broth into a large container or jars using a fine-mesh strainer. Discard the bay leaves, peppercorns, and any unwanted vegetables. Store for up to 5 days.

Prep Tip: If you don't have an Instant Pot, use a large pot and cook on the stovetop—but you'll need more time for the chicken to cook through. Combine all the ingredients in the pot, cover, and cook over high heat, letting the mixture come to a rolling boil, about 20 minutes. Then reduce the heat to medium-low and allow the mixture to simmer for 1 to 3 hours, adding water a cup at a time to ensure the chicken cooks through and plenty of broth is left behind.

Substitution Tip: If you have IBS or Fibromyalgia, replace the garlic and onion with the green portions of 1 bunch of scallions, rinsed.

Per serving: Calories: 158; Total fat: 3g; Carbohydrates: 5g; Fiber: 1g; Protein: 25g; Calcium: 29mg; Vitamin D: 13mcg; Vitamin B12: 0mcg; Iron: 1mg; Zinc: 1mg

Kabocha Squash Soup

Serves 8 / **Prep time: 10 mins** / **Cook time: 35 mins**

DAIRY-FREE   GLUTEN-FREE   NUT-FREE   SOY-FREE

HYPOGLYCEMIA POWER FOOD, INSOMNIA, BRAIN FOG, LOW-FODMAP FOR IBS, MOOD BOOSTER, HASHIMOTO'S POWER FOOD, FIBROMYALGIA POWER FOOD, TOXIN BUSTER

Oven-roasted kabocha squash can be added to salads or grain bowls, eaten as a side, or made into a delicious pureed soup. The nutrients in kabocha squash are perfect for addressing adrenal fatigue—it is high in vitamin A, vitamin C, and magnesium.

1 medium kabocha squash, halved and seeded

1 tablespoon extra-virgin olive oil

2 tablespoons grated fresh ginger

1 tablespoon minced garlic (optional) ◆ / ■

1 teaspoon ground cumin

½ teaspoon ground coriander

¼ teaspoon freshly ground black pepper

3 cups unsalted chicken or vegetable stock

1. Preheat the oven to 425°F and line a large rimmed baking sheet with parchment paper.

2. Put the kabocha squash halves on the prepared baking sheet and roast for 25 to 30 minutes, or until the flesh softens.

3. While the kabocha squash is roasting, heat the olive oil in a large stock-pot over medium-high heat. Add the ginger, garlic, cumin, coriander, and black pepper. Sauté for 2 minutes. Add the stock and bring to a boil.

4. Once the squash is cool enough to handle, use a spoon to scrape the flesh into a blender.

5. Transfer the kabocha flesh to a blender, add the stock and blend until smooth. Serve immediately or cool before storing. Keep refrigerated or freeze for up to 3 months.

Substitution Tip: If you have IBS or Fibromyalgia, omit the garlic, and use garlic-infused oil if desired.

Per serving: Calories: 66; Total fat: 2g; Carbohydrates: 13g; Fiber: 2g; Protein: 1g; Calcium: 40mg; Vitamin D: 0mcg; Vitamin B12: 0mcg; Iron: 1mg; Zinc: 0mg

Lazy Day Italian Wedding Soup

Serves 4 / Prep time: 5 mins / Cook time: 20 mins

DAIRY-FREE   GLUTEN-FREE   NUT-FREE   SOY-FREE

HYPOGLYCEMIA POWER FOOD, INSOMNIA, BRAIN FOG, LOW-FODMAP FOR IBS, MOOD BOOSTER, HASHIMOTO'S POWER FOOD, FIBROMYALGIA POWER FOOD

A really flavorful soup doesn't have to take hours to make—all you need is the right spices and good stock. The meatballs in this recipe are made of the same mixture used in Best Turkey Burgers (page 117), though this soup is still hearty and delicious when made meat-free.

4 cups unsalted chicken stock

1 cup water

½ cup (½ batch) mixture from Best Turkey Burgers (page 117, step 1) ◆ / ■

1 cup rainbow chard, coarsely chopped

1 cup cooked brown rice or quinoa

1 large egg, beaten

Kosher salt

Freshly ground black pepper

½ cup fresh parsley, coarsely chopped, for garnish

1. In a medium saucepan, combine the chicken stock and water and bring to a boil over high heat, about 10 minutes. While the chicken stock is heating, prepare the mixture from Best Turkey Burgers (step 1 only).

2. Make mini meatballs, using about ½ tablespoon of the mixture for each meatball. As you make the meatballs, drop them into the boiling broth and let them cook as you go, for about 5 minutes.

3. Add the rainbow chard and let it wilt for 1 to 2 minutes. Add the rice.

4. Once the soup reaches a rolling boil, slowly drizzle in the egg. Cook for 1 minute. Remove from the heat and add salt and pepper to taste. Garnish with the parsley.

Substitution Tip: If you have IBS or Fibromyalgia, omit the meatballs and enjoy a vegetarian version, or make the adjustments for IBS in the Substitution Tip of the recipe for Best Turkey Burgers (page 117).

Per serving: Calories: 122; Total fat: 4g; Carbohydrates: 15g; Fiber: 1g; Protein: 6g; Calcium: 32mg; Vitamin D: 12mcg; Vitamin B12: 0mcg; Iron: 1mg; Zinc: 1mg

Roasted Vegetable Chili

Serves 8 / Prep time: 10 mins / Cook time: 30 mins

DAIRY-FREE GLUTEN-FREE NUT-FREE SOY-FREE

HYPOGLYCEMIA POWER FOOD, INSOMNIA, BRAIN FOG, MOOD BOOSTER, TOXIN BUSTER

Many of my clients make a large batch of chili to eat throughout the week. Some of them use a lot of red meat—so I created this vegetarian recipe to encourage them to continue their meal prep routine while reducing their red meat intake. This chili uses kidney beans, which have a deep flavor and a meaty texture. If you don't have an Instant Pot, see the Prep Tip after the recipe for stovetop instructions.

½ medium onion, diced ✦ / ■
1 large sweet potato, cut into
  1-inch dice
1 medium zucchini, cut into
  1-inch dice
1 quart unsalted vegetable stock
2 bay leaves
1 teaspoon freshly ground
  black pepper
1 tablespoon ground cumin
1 teaspoon chili powder ●

2 teaspoons dried oregano
1 tablespoon tomato paste ●
1 (15-ounce) can unsalted black
  beans, rinsed and drained
1 (15-ounce) can unsalted kidney
  beans, rinsed and drained
1 (28-ounce) can unsalted diced
  roasted tomatoes ●
½ cup chopped fresh parsley or
  cilantro, for garnish

1. In the bowl of an Instant Pot or other pressure cooker, combine the onion, sweet potato, zucchini, vegetable stock, bay leaves, pepper, cumin, chili powder, oregano, tomato paste, black beans, kidney beans, and diced roasted tomatoes (with their juices). Press the Bean/Chili setting (high pressure), allow it to pressurize, and cook for 30 minutes.

2. Serve hot, garnished with the fresh parsley. Refrigerate leftovers for up to 1 week.

Prep Tip: If you don't have an Instant Pot, use a large pot and cook on the stovetop over medium-high heat. Sauté the onion in 1 tablespoon of olive oil for 2 to 3 minutes, or until translucent. Then add the rest of the ingredients, reduce the heat to medium, and cook, stirring occasionally, for 30 minutes, or until the chili is thickened and the vegetables are tender.

Substitution Tip: If you have Hashimoto's, omit the chili powder and tomato paste and replace the roasted tomatoes with additional vegetable stock. If you have IBS or Fibromyalgia, replace the onion with the green portions of 1 or 2 scallions.

Per serving: Calories: 135; Total fat: 1g; Carbohydrates: 26g; Fiber: 8g; Protein: 8g; Calcium: 81mg; Vitamin D: 0mcg; Vitamin B12: 0mcg; Iron: 3mg; Zinc: 1mg

30-Minute Chicken Pho

Serves 4 / Prep time: 5 mins / Cook time: 25 mins

DAIRY-FREE   GLUTEN-FREE   NUT-FREE   SOY-FREE

INSOMNIA, MOOD BOOSTER, HASHIMOTO'S POWER FOOD,
FIBROMYALGIA POWER FOOD, TOXIN BUSTER

This is one of my favorite recipes to make. I'm not usually a fan of replacing wheat or rice noodles with vegetable noodles, but the zucchini noodles in this recipe work perfectly and absorb a ton of flavor. If you have cooked chicken and spiralized zucchini in the refrigerator and chicken broth in the pantry, you can have this delicious dinner ready in less than 10 minutes!

8 cups unsalted chicken broth

1 bunch fresh cilantro, stems and leaves separated

1 tablespoon minced fresh ginger

5 garlic cloves, smashed ◆ / ▣

4 cups water

2 large boneless, skinless chicken breasts (about 4 ounces each)

1 small onion, thinly sliced ◆ / ▣

Juice of 1½ limes

2 tablespoons coconut aminos

2 tablespoons pure maple syrup (skip for Week 3, Week 4, and the Flare-Up Meal Plan)

4 cups spiralized zucchini, for serving

1 cup fresh basil, for garnish

2 cups bean sprouts, for garnish

1. In a large pot, combine the chicken broth, cilantro stems, ginger, garlic, and water and bring to a boil over high heat.

2. Add the chicken breasts and onion and cook for 15 to 20 minutes, or until the chicken is cooked through.

3. Remove the chicken breasts and shred the meat with a fork.

4. Add the lime juice, coconut aminos, and maple syrup to the broth and boil for 5 minutes.

5. If serving immediately, ladle 1½ cups of the hot broth into each of 4 large soup bowls and add 1 cup of spiralized zucchini and ½ cup of the shredded chicken to each bowl. Garnish with the basil, cilantro leaves, and bean sprouts. If storing, keep the zucchini and garnishes separate and store the shredded chicken in the broth to retain moisture.

Stretch Tip: Leftover chicken is great on salad, in warm grain bowls, or with vegetable sides to make a complete meal. Use leftover leaves from the cilantro in another recipe, like the Peruvian Green Spicy Sauce (page 147).

Substitution Tip: If you have IBS or Fibromyalgia, replace the garlic and onion with the green portions of 2 or 3 scallions.

Per serving: Calories: 229; Total fat: 3g; Carbohydrates: 31g; Fiber: 5g; Protein: 24g; Calcium: 112mg; Vitamin D: 8mcg; Vitamin B12: Omcg; Iron: 3mg; Zinc: 2mg

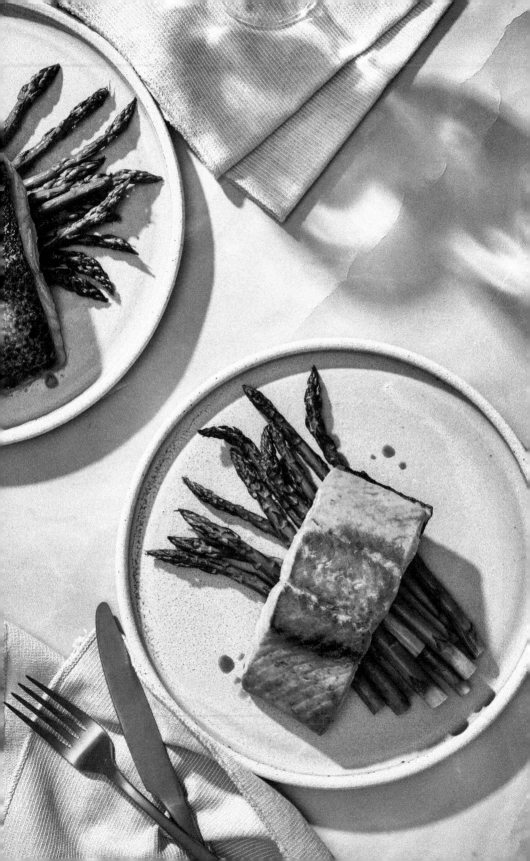

Chapter 8

Dinner Mains

Baked Mustard Salmon

Serves 4 / Prep time: 5 mins / Cook time: 15 mins

DAIRY-FREE   GLUTEN-FREE   NUT-FREE   SOY-FREE

INSOMNIA, BRAIN FOG, LOW-FODMAP FOR IBS, MOOD BOOSTER, HASHIMOTO'S POWER FOOD, FIBROMYALGIA POWER FOOD

This is my go-to menu item for a dinner party. It's simple to make, and it's a crowd-pleaser. For my clients who are not vegan or vegetarian, I recommend eating fish two or three times per week. Salmon is one of the most nutrient-dense foods available and an excellent source of omega-3 fatty acids, vitamin D, and B vitamins, which are all vital to adrenal health. This salmon pairs well with any of the sides in chapter 9 (page 127).

2 tablespoons Dijon mustard
1 tablespoon pure maple syrup (skip for Week 3, Week 4, and the Flare-Up Meal Plan)

2 tablespoons extra-virgin olive oil
1½ pounds wild Atlantic salmon
⅛ teaspoon kosher salt

1. Preheat the oven to 375°F. Line a rimmed baking sheet with parchment paper.

2. In a small bowl, combine the mustard, maple syrup, and olive oil.

3. Put the salmon on the prepared baking sheet and spread the mustard sauce evenly across it. Sprinkle with the salt.

4. Bake the salmon for about 15 minutes, or until cooked through. Serve hot or cold. Refrigerate for up to 3 days. If serving later, reheat the salmon in the oven at 275°F for 15 minutes.

Prep Tip: If you don't like the idea of reheating cooked fish, add cold salmon to any salad, grain bowls, or even fried rice.

Substitution Tip: If wild Atlantic salmon is not available, try ethically farmed King or Coho salmon (see SeafoodWatch.org for more information).

Per serving: Calories: 319; Total fat: 18g; Carbohydrates: 4g; Fiber: 0g; Protein: 34g; Calcium: 30mg; Vitamin D: 434mcg; Vitamin B12: 5mcg; Iron: 2mg; Zinc: 1mg

Best Turkey Burgers

Serves 4 / **Prep time: 10 mins** / **Cook time: 10 mins**

DAIRY-FREE   GLUTEN-FREE   NUT-FREE   SOY-FREE

INSOMNIA, LOW-FODMAP FOR IBS, MOOD BOOSTER, HASHIMOTO'S POWER FOOD, FIBROMYALGIA POWER FOOD, TOXIN BUSTER

Until this recipe came along, I thought all turkey burgers were dry and flavorless. Shredded zucchini provides moisture, making these burgers juicy, delicious, and full of fiber. Spices and mint add a burst of flavor. I like to panfry mini burgers for grain bowls, salads, or lettuce wraps and use leftover mixture in meatballs for Lazy Day Italian Wedding Soup (page 109). I challenge you to use part of this recipe in a different dish!

1 pound ground turkey
1 medium zucchini, shredded
1 scallion, green and white parts, finely chopped ◆ / ■
1 large egg, beaten

6 fresh mint leaves, minced
2 garlic cloves, minced ◆ / ■
¼ cup fresh cilantro, finely chopped
1 tablespoon ground cumin
2 tablespoons extra-virgin olive oil

1. In a large bowl, combine the ground turkey, zucchini, scallion, egg, mint, garlic, cilantro, and cumin and stir well to incorporate.

2. Shape the ground turkey mixture into 2- to 3-inch balls. Flatten gently into patties.

3. Heat the olive oil in a large nonstick skillet over medium heat. Fry the patties for about 2 minutes on each side, or until browned and crispy.

Stretch Tip: Save a third to half of the burger mix, and use it to make mini meatballs for Lazy Day Italian Wedding Soup (page 109), Shakshuka (page 80), or any other soup or sauce.

Substitution Tip: If you have IBS or Fibromyalgia, use only the green portion of the scallion (not the white), and omit the garlic.

Per serving: Calories: 261; Total fat: 17g; Carbohydrates: 3g; Fiber: 1g; Protein: 25g; Calcium: 53mg; Vitamin D: 25mcg; Vitamin B12: 1mcg; Iron: 3mg; Zinc: 3mg

Warm Green Lentil Salad

Serves 4 / Prep time: 5 mins, plus lentil cooking time / Cook time: less than 5 mins

DAIRY-FREE GLUTEN-FREE NUT-FREE SOY-FREE

HYPOGLYCEMIA POWER FOOD, INSOMNIA, LOW-FODMAP FOR IBS, MOOD BOOSTER, HASHIMOTO'S POWER FOOD, FIBROMYALGIA POWER FOOD, TOXIN BUSTER

Lentils are delicious and packed with nutrients. They are high in fiber, which can help your body regulate its blood sugar levels. They are also a great source of prebiotics, which support good gut health. If you have cooked lentils ready, this salad takes less than 10 minutes to prepare—purchasing canned or vacuum-packed cooked lentils can save you lots of time.

1½ cups canned or cooked unsalted green or brown lentils
2 cups baby arugula
5 fresh mint leaves, finely chopped
2 tablespoons chopped fresh cilantro

1 small shallot, finely chopped ◆ / ▣
¼ cup Dijon Mustard Vinaigrette (page 151)
4 large eggs
Extra-virgin olive oil, for frying

1. Put the cooked lentils in a large microwave-safe bowl and microwave (at 1,200 watts) for 2 to 3 minutes, or until warmed through.

2. Add the arugula, mint, cilantro, and shallot and stir to incorporate.

3. Drizzle the mixture with the vinaigrette and mix well to combine.

4. In a small nonstick skillet, fry the eggs in olive oil over medium-high heat for 2 to 3 minutes, or to your preference. Top the lentil salad with the fried eggs and serve hot or cold.

Prep Tip: If you're taking this salad to go, skip step 3 and store the dressing on the side so that the salad doesn't get soggy.

Substitution Tip: If you have IBS or Fibromyalgia, omit the shallot.

Per serving: Calories: 243; Total fat: 15g; Carbohydrates: 16g; Fiber: 6g; Protein: 13g; Calcium: 56mg; Vitamin D: 36mcg; Vitamin B12: 0mcg; Iron: 3mg; Zinc: 2mg

Roasted Eggplant Ragù

Serves 6 / Prep time: 5 mins / Cook time: 35 mins

DAIRY-FREE   GLUTEN-FREE   NUT-FREE   SOY-FREE

INSOMNIA, MOOD BOOSTER, BRAIN FOG, TOXIN BUSTER

Many of my clients have told me that they love eggplants but find them difficult to cook with. When eggplants are oven-roasted correctly, they're delicious enough to eat straight out of the oven—and with a hearty tomato sauce, they're even better. Use the leftover tomato sauce from this recipe in Shakshuka (page 80).

1 large eggplant, cut into 1-inch dice

4 tablespoons extra-virgin olive oil, divided

2 garlic cloves, minced ◆ / ■

1 shallot, chopped ◆ / ■

10 to 12 button mushrooms, cut into small pieces

1 (15-ounce) can crushed tomatoes

16 ounces tomato sauce

1 cup chopped fresh parsley

5 fresh basil leaves (optional)

3 cups cooked whole grains of your choice (optional), **for serving**

1. Preheat the oven to 425°F and line a large rimmed baking sheet with parchment paper.

2. Put the eggplant on the prepared baking sheet, drizzle with 2 tablespoons of olive oil, and toss to coat. Spread the eggplant into a single layer and roast for 20 minutes, or until the edges are browning.

3. While the eggplant roasts, make the tomato sauce. Heat the remaining 2 tablespoons of olive oil in a large skillet over medium-high heat. Add the garlic and shallot and sauté for about 3 minutes, or until translucent.

4. Add the mushrooms and sauté for 3 minutes, or until softened. Pour in the crushed tomatoes and tomato sauce, reduce the heat to medium, and cook for about 10 minutes, stirring occasionally, to allow the mixture to thicken.

continued »

5. Transfer the roasted eggplant to the skillet. Add the parsley and basil (if using) and cook for 5 minutes, or until softened and fragrant. Serve plain or over ½ cup whole grain of your choice.

Substitution Tip: If you have IBS or Fibromyalgia, omit the garlic and shallot and use garlic-infused olive oil.

Per serving: Calories: 141; Total fat: 10g; Carbohydrates: 14g; Fiber: 6g; Protein: 3g; Calcium: 58mg; Vitamin D: 1mcg; Vitamin B12: 0mcg; Iron: 2mg; Zinc: 1mg

Shrimp Tacos with Black Bean Salad

Serves 4 / **Prep time: 5 mins** / **Cook time: 15 mins**

DAIRY-FREE   GLUTEN-FREE   NUT-FREE   SOY-FREE

HYPONATREMIA, INSOMNIA, BRAIN FOG, MOOD BOOSTER,
HASHIMOTO'S POWER FOOD, TOXIN BUSTER

Traditional tacos are made with flour or corn tortillas, but even if you're avoiding those ingredients, you don't need to miss out on good tacos! This recipe uses butter lettuce leaves instead of tortillas—they're the perfect round shape!—but you can also use thin lentil or buckwheat pancakes.

For the shrimp
2 tablespoons extra-virgin olive oil
2 garlic cloves, minced ◆ / ■
1 teaspoon grated fresh ginger
1½ pounds wild shrimp, peeled
  and deveined
⅛ teaspoon kosher salt

⅛ teaspoon freshly ground
  black pepper
1 tablespoon freshly squeezed
  lemon juice
2 tablespoons chopped fresh parsley
  or cilantro

For the black bean salad
1 (15-ounce) can black beans, drained
  and rinsed
1 medium tomato, chopped ●
1 small to medium shallot, finely
  chopped ◆ / ■

Juice of 1 lime
Kosher salt
Freshly ground black pepper

For the tacos
½ cup Quick Pickled Red Onions
  (page 150) ◆
1 avocado, pitted and thinly sliced

2 heads butter lettuce (about
  20 large outer leaves)
1 lime, cut into wedges

1. **To make the shrimp:** Heat the olive oil in a large nonstick skillet over medium-high heat. Add the garlic and ginger and sauté for 1 minute, or until fragrant. Add the shrimp, salt, and pepper and cook for 2 to 3 minutes on each side, stirring occasionally, or until the shrimp are pink and opaque. Drizzle with the lemon juice, sprinkle with the parsley or cilantro, and set aside.

continued ››

2. **To make the black bean salad:** In a medium mixing bowl, combine the black beans, tomato, shallot, and lime juice. Season with salt and pepper. Toss well.

3. **To make the tacos:** Make your own tacos with the bean salad, shrimp, pickled red onions, and avocado on butter lettuce. Serve with the lime wedges.

Prep Tip: This recipe can be made with leftover chicken or made fully vegetarian. To make it ahead, prepare the shrimp, black bean salad, and Quick Pickled Red Onions and refrigerate for up to 3 days; then assemble just before serving. This recipe is also easy to scale up for a large party.

Substitution Tip: If you have Hashimoto's, replace the tomatoes with radishes. If you have **IBS** or **Fibromyalgia**, omit the shallot, replace the garlic with the green portions of 1 or 2 scallions, and skip the Quick Pickled Red Onions.

Per serving: Calories: 384; Total fat: 17g; Carbohydrates: 29g; Fiber: 11g; Protein: 32g; Calcium: 158mg; Vitamin D: 3mcg; Vitamin B12: 2mcg; Iron: 3mg; Zinc: 3mg

Crispy Chicken Tenders

Serves 4 / **Prep time: 5 mins** / **Cook time: 20 mins**

DAIRY-FREE   GLUTEN-FREE   SOY-FREE

INSOMNIA, MOOD BOOSTER, HASHIMOTO'S POWER FOOD,
TOXIN BUSTER

Chicken tenders aren't just for kids! Rather than coating these with heavy white flour and bread crumbs, I use a mixture of seeds. Seeds add fiber, vitamins, and minerals that are great for your adrenal health, and they also give these chicken tenders a crispy exterior. These are so flavorful that they don't need a dipping sauce, but if you want one, Creamy Tahini Dressing (page 146) and Peruvian Green Spicy Sauce (page 147) both work well.

1 teaspoon kosher salt
1 cup almond flour ◆
2 teaspoons garlic powder ◆ / ■
1 cup chia seeds
½ cup sesame seeds
1 cup flaxseed

2 large eggs
1 cup potato starch ●
4 tablespoons olive oil or coconut oil, divided, for frying
1 pound chicken breast tenders, pounded to ½-inch thickness

1. In a shallow dish, combine the salt, almond flour, garlic powder, chia seeds, sesame seeds, and flaxseed. Stir to combine.

2. In a second shallow dish, beat the eggs. Put the potato starch in a third shallow dish.

3. Heat 2 tablespoons of olive oil in a large nonstick skillet over medium-high heat.

4. Coat your chicken tenders one at a time. First dip them in the potato starch, next in the eggs, and then in the seed and almond flour mixture, pressing well to coat.

5. Add the breaded chicken tenders to the skillet, a few at a time, and cook for about 4 minutes on each side, or until golden brown. Slice 1 tender to ensure it has cooked through. Repeat with the remaining 2 tablespoons of olive oil and the rest of the chicken tenders. Serve hot or cool before storing.

continued »

Prep Tip: You can also bake these chicken tenders in the oven at 350°F for 20 minutes. Line a rimmed baking sheet with parchment paper, and spray the chicken tenders with cooking oil before baking. For meal prep purposes, double this recipe to make a larger batch, and reheat the chicken tenders at 275°F for 15 minutes.

Substitution Tip: If you have IBS or Fibromyalgia, omit the garlic powder (you can add another seasoning of your choice, such as lemon pepper), and if you have IBS, use oat flour instead of almond flour. If you have Hashimoto's, replace the potato starch with additional almond flour.

Per serving: Calories: 360; Total fat: 20g; Carbohydrates: 15g; Fiber: 6g; Protein: 31g; Calcium: 105mg; Vitamin D: 11mcg; Vitamin B12: 0mcg; Iron: 2mg; Zinc: 2mg

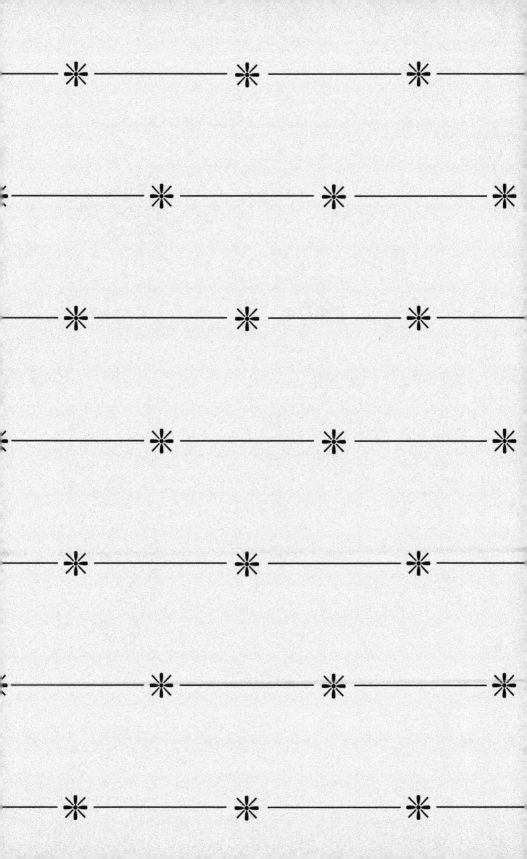

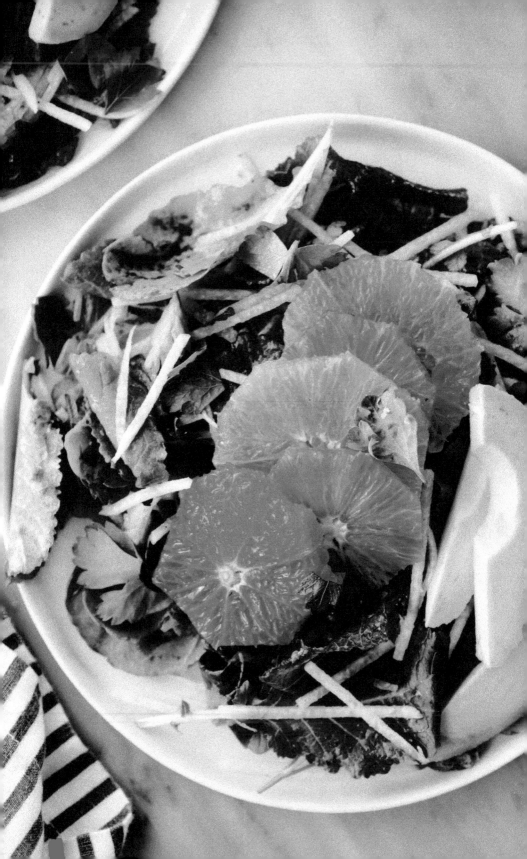

Chapter 9

Salads and Sides

Cilantro-Lime Rice

Serves 4 / Prep time: 5 mins / Cook time: 25 mins (or 5 mins if using precooked rice)

DAIRY-FREE   GLUTEN-FREE   NUT-FREE   SOY-FREE

HYPOGLYCEMIA POWER FOOD, BRAIN FOG, LOW-FODMAP FOR IBS, MOOD BOOSTER, HASHIMOTO'S POWER FOOD, FIBROMYALGIA POWER FOOD, TOXIN BUSTER

I grew up eating plain white rice as my main source of carbohydrates. Since white rice is not a whole grain, we'll use brown rice in this dish. Cilantro-lime rice is perfect on its own or served with roasted chicken and vegetables. I love to use this recipe to turn my leftover rice into something interesting and flavorful. It's delicious served warm or cold.

1½ cups water
1 cup uncooked brown rice (or 2 cups
   leftover cooked brown rice)
½ cup fresh cilantro
Juice of 1 lime

1 tablespoon extra-virgin olive oil
1 garlic clove ◆ / ■
Salt
Freshly ground black pepper

1. In a small saucepan, bring the water to a boil over high heat. Add the rice, cover with a lid, reduce the heat to medium-low, and simmer for about 20 minutes, or until the water is absorbed and the rice is tender. (If using leftover cooked rice, microwave for about 2 minutes, or until warm.)

2. While the rice cooks, in a food processor, combine the cilantro, lime juice, olive oil, and garlic.

3. Add the cilantro-lime mixture to the cooked rice and fluff with a fork to combine. Add salt and pepper to taste. Serve hot or refrigerate leftovers for up to 4 days.

Substitution Tip: If you have IBS or Fibromyalgia, replace the garlic with the green portion of 1 scallion.

Per serving: Calories: 206; Total fat: 5g; Carbohydrates: 37g; Fiber: 2g; Protein: 4g; Calcium: 20mg; Vitamin D: 0mcg; Vitamin B12: 0mcg; Iron: 1mg; Zinc: 1mg

Roasted Sweet Potato "Hummus"

Serves 8 to 10 / Prep time: 5 mins / Cook time: 25 mins, plus cooling

DAIRY-FREE   GLUTEN-FREE   NUT-FREE   SOY-FREE

HYPOGLYCEMIA POWER FOOD, LOW-FODMAP FOR IBS, MOOD
BOOSTER, HASHIMOTO'S POWER FOOD, FIBROMYALGIA POWER FOOD,
TOXIN BUSTER

One of my favorite vegetarian restaurants in New York City, NIX, serves
the most delicious and creative dips I have ever tasted. Inspired by them,
I developed this recipe to enjoy at home. This "hummus" pairs well with
seed crackers, vegetable crudités, and wraps. When I roast vegetables for
the week, I sometimes include extra sweet potatoes to have ready for this
recipe—then I can throw it together in less than 5 minutes!

2 large sweet potatoes, cut into 1- to
 1½-inch dice
3 garlic cloves ◆ / ▦
2 tablespoons extra-virgin olive oil

6 tablespoons tahini
Juice of 1 small lime
⅛ teaspoon kosher salt
1 cup water

1. Preheat the oven to 400°F. Line a rimmed baking sheet with
    parchment paper.

2. Put the sweet potatoes and garlic cloves on the prepared baking sheet
    and drizzle with the olive oil, tossing to coat. Roast for 20 minutes, or
    until lightly browned and tender when pierced.

3. Let the roasted sweet potatoes and garlic cool and then combine with
    the tahini, lime juice, salt, and water in an upright blender. Puree the
    mixture until creamy. Serve warm or refrigerate for 1 hour before serving.
    Refrigerate leftovers for up to 4 days.

Substitution Tip: If you have IBS or Fibromyalgia, omit the garlic and
use garlic-infused olive oil in place of regular olive oil. Or omit the garlic
altogether—this recipe is delicious either way.

Per serving: Calories: 128; Total fat: 9g; Carbohydrates: 10g; Fiber: 2g; Protein: 2g;
Calcium: 61mg; Vitamin D: 0mcg; Vitamin B12: 0mcg; Iron: 1mg; Zinc: 1mg

Sautéed Broccoli with Raisins

Serves 4 / **Prep time: 10 mins** / **Cook time: 10 mins**

DAIRY-FREE   GLUTEN-FREE   NUT-FREE   SOY-FREE

INSOMNIA, LOW-FODMAP FOR IBS, BRAIN FOG, MOOD BOOSTER, FIBROMYALGIA POWER FOOD, TOXIN BUSTER

I always tell my clients to explore outside of the entrée section of the menu when they go out to eat, and they're often pleasantly surprised to find that many side dishes steal the show and can be eaten as entrées. This broccoli dish is inspired by similar side dishes at some of my favorite Italian restaurants in California and New York City. It's rich, is slightly sweet, and has a nice crunch. Sometimes I like to top it with two soft-boiled eggs to make it feel like a complete meal.

2 tablespoons extra-virgin olive oil

1 head broccoli, cut into florets with long stems

2 tablespoons raisins

2 tablespoons chicken broth or vegetable broth

⅛ teaspoon kosher salt

⅛ teaspoon freshly ground black pepper

3 tablespoons Creamy Tahini Dressing (page 146), **for serving**

1 teaspoon sumac, **for serving**

1. Heat the olive oil in a large pan or cast-iron skillet over medium heat. Add the broccoli and cook for about 5 minutes, turning the pieces occasionally to ensure even cooking, or until the broccoli is bright green and slightly tender.

2. Add the raisins, broth, salt, and pepper and cook for 1 to 2 minutes.

3. To serve, transfer the hot broccoli to a dish, drizzle with the Creamy Tahini Dressing, and sprinkle with the sumac.

A Closer Look: Sumac is a Middle Eastern spice made from dried and ground berries with a unique citrusy flavor that pairs well with roasted vegetables, salads, and chicken. Sumac is also a powerful anti-inflammatory that can help neutralize free radicals in your body. If you can't find sumac, you can use lemon zest and salt instead.

Per serving: Calories: 162; Total fat: 12g; Carbohydrates: 11g; Fiber: 4g; Protein: 4g; Calcium: 89mg; Vitamin D: 0mcg; Vitamin B12: 0mcg; Iron: 1mg; Zinc: 1mg

Roasted Summer Vegetables

Serves 6 / Prep time: 10 mins / Cook time: 30 mins

DAIRY-FREE GLUTEN-FREE NUT-FREE SOY-FREE

HYPOGLYCEMIA POWER FOOD, BRAIN FOG, MOOD BOOSTER,
HASHIMOTO'S POWER FOOD, FIBROMYALGIA POWER FOOD,
TOXIN BUSTER

When fresh fruits and vegetables are in season, they don't require much seasoning for the flavors to pop. This recipe puts vegetables front and center, seasoned with just olive oil, salt, pepper, and herbes de Provence. I encourage my clients to roast one big batch of vegetables at once and use them for quick meals all week long—like in grain bowls, in soups, or as a side.

1 large delicata squash, halved, seeded, and cut into 1-inch half-moons ◆ / ■
1 large zucchini, cut into thick rounds
5 roma tomatoes, quartered, or 1 pint cherry tomatoes ●

2 tablespoons extra-virgin olive oil
1 tablespoon herbes de Provence
⅛ teaspoon kosher salt
⅛ teaspoon freshly ground black pepper

1. Preheat the oven to 400°F. Line a rimmed baking sheet with parchment paper.

2. Put the squash, zucchini, and tomatoes on the prepared baking sheet, drizzle with the olive oil, and sprinkle with the herbes de Provence, salt, and pepper. Toss the mixture to coat and spread into a single layer.

3. Bake the vegetables for 30 minutes, flipping the squash and zucchini halfway through, or until the squash and zucchini are browned and the tomatoes are juicy. Serve warm or allow to cool and refrigerate for up to 5 days.

Prep Tip: Tomatoes can release a lot of juice during the baking process, so it's best to keep them separate from the zucchini and squash.

Substitution Tip: If you have IBS or Fibromyalgia, use kabocha squash instead of delicata. If you have Hashimoto's, omit the tomatoes.

Per serving: Calories: 80; Total fat: 5g; Carbohydrates: 10g; Fiber: 2g; Protein: 1g; Calcium: 34mg; Vitamin D: 0mcg; Vitamin B12: 0mcg; Iron: 1mg; Zinc: 0mg

Roasted Beet Salad with Orange and Avocado

Serves 4 / Prep time: 10 mins

DAIRY-FREE GLUTEN-FREE SOY-FREE

HYPOGLYCEMIA POWER FOOD, BRAIN FOG, MOOD BOOSTER, HASHIMOTO'S POWER FOOD, TOXIN BUSTER

Beets are delicious and packed with so many nutrients that play important roles in addressing adrenal fatigue symptoms. One of these nutrients is folate, which is crucial to proper cellular, neurological, and nervous system function. The one downside to beets is their long cooking time, but you can find precooked beets at most supermarkets.

5 to 7 whole precooked beets, cut into bite-size pieces (2 to 3 cups)

1 large orange, peeled and cut into half-moons

⅛ cup raw or roasted and unsalted pine nuts

⅛ teaspoon kosher salt

⅛ teaspoon freshly ground black pepper

1 tablespoon sherry vinegar

¼ cup extra-virgin olive oil

3 cups baby arugula

1 avocado, pitted and thinly sliced

In a large salad bowl, combine the beets, orange, pine nuts, salt, pepper, sherry vinegar, olive oil, arugula, and avocado and toss to coat.

Substitution Tip: If you can't find pine nuts, you can use chopped pistachios, hazelnuts, or even walnuts, depending on your preference.

Prep Tip: If you can't find precooked beets, boil raw beets in a saucepan for 30 to 40 minutes, or until tender. Allow them to cool before peeling and slicing them. This salad is best served fresh, but if you're eating it later, add the avocado and arugula just before serving.

Per serving: Calories: 314; Total fat: 25g; Carbohydrates: 23g; Fiber: 9g; Protein: 5g; Calcium: 68mg; Vitamin D: 0mcg; Vitamin B12: 0mcg; Iron: 2mg; Zinc: 1mg

Simple Base Salad

Serves 6 / Prep time: 10 mins

DAIRY-FREE   GLUTEN-FREE   SOY-FREE

LOW-FODMAP FOR IBS, BRAIN FOG, MOOD BOOSTER, FIBROMYALGIA
POWER FOOD, TOXIN BUSTER

When building a well-balanced salad, think 50 percent leafy greens, 25 percent non-starchy vegetables, 15 percent lean protein (whole grains, beans, fish, chicken, and turkey) or starchy vegetables, and 10 percent plant-based fat (oils, nuts, and avocado). Plain salad greens are healthy, but they lack fiber and the calories needed for a full meal—you'll be hungry again in an hour. Use this salad as a starting point and add whatever fresh vegetables or protein you have on hand.

4 cups baby spinach
2 cups baby arugula
1 small orange, sliced
5 radishes, thinly sliced
1 cup diced seedless cucumber
1 cup torn fresh herbs of your
   choice, such as basil, cilantro,
   parsley, or mint

¼ cup chopped roasted unsalted nuts
   of your choice
¼ cup Dijon Mustard Vinaigrette
   (page 151)

In a large salad bowl, combine the spinach, arugula, oranges, radishes, cucumber, and herbs. When ready to serve, toss with the nuts and vinaigrette.

Prep Tip: If you're meal-prepping this salad to eat later, combine all the ingredients except the nuts and vinaigrette. If you wash any ingredients, make sure to dry them before adding them to the salad to prevent wilting. Store the nuts and vinaigrette separately.

Per serving: Calories: 113; Total fat: 11g; Carbohydrates: 4g; Fiber: 2g; Protein: 2g; Calcium: 62mg; Vitamin D: 0mcg; Vitamin B12: 0mcg; Iron: 2mg; Zinc: 0mg

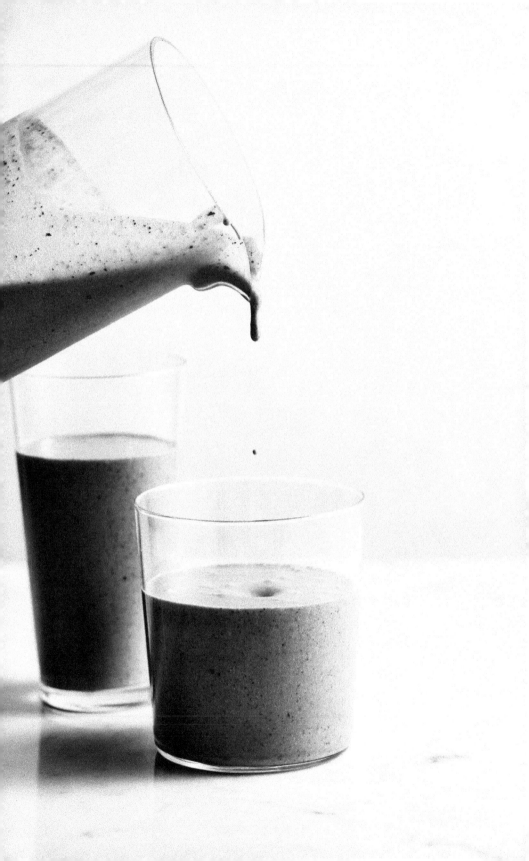

Chapter 10

Sweet Treats

Chocolate Energy Bites

Serves 8 to 10 (makes 16 to 20 energy bites) / **Prep time: 15 mins, plus 30 mins refrigeration**

DAIRY-FREE GLUTEN-FREE SOY-FREE

HYPOGLYCEMIA POWER FOOD, LOW-FODMAP FOR IBS, BRAIN FOG, HASHIMOTO'S POWER FOOD, FIBROMYALGIA POWER FOOD, MOOD BOOSTER, TOXIN BUSTER

I first made these energy bites as pre- and post-run fuel while my husband was training for a marathon. My son absolutely loved these as a snack with a cold glass of oat milk. Now this is everyone's favorite snack in my house. The recipe is easy to make—no baking required—and the energy bites keep well in the refrigerator. Make a batch over the weekend to last you for a few weeks.

1 cup gluten-free rolled oats
6 medjool dates
2 tablespoons unsweetened
   cocoa powder
6 tablespoons unsalted
   almond butter ◆

2 tablespoons chia seeds
1 tablespoon alcohol- and sugar-free
   vanilla extract
¼ teaspoon vanilla beans (optional)
1 tablespoon hemp seeds (optional)

1. In a food processor, combine the rolled oats, dates, cocoa powder, almond butter, chia seeds, vanilla extract, vanilla beans (if using), and hemp seeds (if using). Pulse for about 1 minute, or until a sticky, coarse dough forms.

2. Scoop out 2 tablespoons of the dough at a time and roll into 1½-inch balls with your hands. Refrigerate in a single layer for at least 30 minutes before serving. Keep the energy bites in the refrigerator for 2 to 3 weeks.

Substitution Tip: If you have IBS, replace the almond butter with peanut butter. If you don't have chia seeds, use flaxseed or hemp seeds (a complete protein) instead.

Per serving: Calories: 224; Total fat: 9g; Carbohydrates: 31g; Fiber: 6g; Protein: 7g; Calcium: 88mg; Vitamin D: 0mcg; Vitamin B12: 0mcg; Iron: 2mg; Zinc: 2mg

Cashew Butter Cups

Serves 12 / Prep time: 15 mins, plus 1 hour 30 mins refrigeration

DAIRY-FREE   GLUTEN-FREE   SOY-FREE

HYPOGLYCEMIA POWER FOOD, LOW-FODMAP FOR IBS, BRAIN FOG, MOOD BOOSTER

When my clients begin following a restrictive diet for their health, the first thing they miss is almost always dessert. Over the years, I have tried my best to find products and create recipes to recommend that are as good as (or better than) the ones they're used to eating. These cashew butter cups are high on my list of recommendations.

1 cup unsalted, unsweetened cashew butter ◆

4 tablespoons pure maple syrup, divided

⅔ cup coconut oil, melted

⅔ cup unsweetened cocoa powder

1 teaspoon coarse sea salt, such as Maldon sea salt flakes

1. Line a 12-cup mini muffin tin with paper liners.

2. In a small bowl, combine the cashew butter and 1 tablespoon of maple syrup. Scoop heaping tablespoons of the mixture into each of the mini muffin cups. Freeze for about 1 hour, or until hardened.

3. While the nut butter mixture is in the freezer, make the chocolate mixture. In a medium mixing bowl, combine the melted coconut oil, cocoa powder, and remaining 3 tablespoons of maple syrup. Stir until smooth.

4. Once the cashew butter mixture is hardened, remove the muffin tin from the freezer and add a tablespoon of the chocolate mixture to each cup to cover the cashew butter mixture. Sprinkle the cashew butter cups with the sea salt and return to the freezer for about 30 minutes, or until the chocolate is hardened.

5. Store the cashew butter cups in the freezer for up to 1 month.

Substitution Tip: If you have IBS, make this recipe with peanut butter instead of cashew butter. If you don't have maple syrup, use honey instead.

Per serving: Calories: 258; Total fat: 23g; Carbohydrates: 13g; Fiber: 2g; Protein: 5g; Calcium: 22mg; Vitamin D: 0mcg; Vitamin B12: 0mcg; Iron: 2mg; Zinc: 2mg

Strawberry-Banana Nice Cream

Serves 2 / Prep time: 5 mins

DAIRY-FREE   GLUTEN-FREE   NUT-FREE   SOY-FREE

HYPOGLYCEMIA POWER FOOD, BRAIN FOG, MOOD BOOSTER,
HASHIMOTO'S POWER FOOD, TOXIN BUSTER

You don't need an ice cream maker for this recipe—just frozen fruit and
a high-speed blender! When my bananas start to get overripe, I peel and
freeze them to use in this recipe. Frozen fruits are often more nutritious
than their fresh counterparts, especially when out of season. This ice
cream won't retain its creamy texture when refrozen, so prepare it just
before serving.

1½ cups frozen strawberries

1 cup frozen ripe banana
(1 or 2 bananas)

In a blender, combine the frozen strawberries and banana. Blend for
30 seconds to 1 minute, or until the mixture has the texture of frozen
yogurt. Transfer to bowls and serve immediately.

Substitution Tip: Bananas can be a base for any flavor of nice cream,
so experiment with different frozen fruits. Try serving with 1 teaspoon of
chopped nuts to add some crunch.

Per serving: Calories: 100; Total fat: 0g; Carbohydrates: 26g; Fiber: 4g; Protein: 1g;
Calcium: 21mg; Vitamin D: 0mcg; Vitamin B12: 0mcg; Iron: 1mg; Zinc: 0mg

Flourless Chickpea Blondies

Serves 12 / Prep time: 10 mins / Cook time: 25 mins

DAIRY-FREE   GLUTEN-FREE   SOY-FREE

HYPOGLYCEMIA POWER FOOD, INSOMNIA, LOW-FODMAP FOR IBS,
BRAIN FOG, MOOD BOOSTER, FIBROMYALGIA POWER FOOD

Don't let the chickpeas in this recipe put you off. When blended into
batter, they make for super moist, delicious blondies with a rich nutty
flavor. This recipe is full of fiber, protein, and healthy fats, a far cry from
the typical sugar-filled blondie recipe. I have been making variations on
this recipe since I was in grad school, so it's an old favorite. Best of all, it's
easy to make—all the ingredients go straight from the food processor to a
baking pan.

½ teaspoon olive oil or coconut oil

1 (15-ounce) can unsalted chickpeas,
rinsed and drained

⅓ cup unsalted, unsweetened
almond butter ◆

¼ cup pure maple syrup

1 tablespoon alcohol- and sugar-free
vanilla extract

¼ teaspoon aluminum-free
baking powder

¼ teaspoon baking soda

¼ teaspoon kosher salt

1. Preheat the oven to 350°F. Grease a 9-by-9-inch baking pan with the oil.

2. In a food processor, combine the chickpeas, almond butter, maple syrup,
   vanilla, baking powder, baking soda, and salt and pulse until a smooth,
   thick batter forms. Transfer the batter to the greased baking pan and
   spread into an even layer.

3. Bake for about 25 minutes, or until a toothpick inserted in the center of
   the blondies comes out clean. Allow to cool completely before cutting
   into 12 squares. Refrigerate the blondies for up to 1 week in an airtight
   container or for up to 1 month in the freezer.

Substitution Tip: If you have IBS, replace the almond butter with
peanut butter.

Per serving: Calories: 98; Total fat: 5g; Carbohydrates: 12g; Fiber: 2g; Protein: 3g;
Calcium: 45mg; Vitamin D: 0mcg; Vitamin B12: 0mcg; Iron: 1mg; Zinc: 1mg

Dark Chocolate Dipper

Serves 4 to 6 / **Prep time: 5 mins, plus 10 mins refrigeration**

DAIRY-FREE   GLUTEN-FREE   NUT-FREE   SOY-FREE

HYPOGLYCEMIA POWER FOOD, LOW-FODMAP FOR IBS, BRAIN FOG, MOOD BOOSTER, FIBROMYALGIA POWER FOOD

For years, I've struggled to find baking chocolate that doesn't contain soy lecithin or refined sugar. I haven't found any yet, so I created this recipe as a rich, luxurious dipping chocolate for my clients to enjoy without worrying about flare-ups. This chocolate is also fantastic drizzled or spread on Flourless Chickpea Blondies (page 139).

⅔ cup coconut oil, melted
⅔ cup unsweetened cocoa powder
⅛ teaspoon kosher salt
¼ cup pure maple syrup

2 cups sliced fresh fruit of your choice, such as berries, pineapple, pears, or apples, for serving

1. In a medium mixing bowl, combine the coconut oil, cocoa powder, salt, and maple syrup. Stir until the chocolate is smooth and no lumps remain.

2. Refrigerate the chocolate for about 10 minutes, or until thickened slightly. Serve with the sliced fresh fruit for dipping.

3. Refrigerate any leftover chocolate dipper for up to 2 weeks.

Prep Tip: Because of the coconut oil, leftover chocolate dipper sauce will harden completely. Rather than reheating it in the microwave, remove it from the refrigerator an hour before you plan to serve it and let it soften at room temperature.

Per serving: Calories: 281; Total fat: 25g; Carbohydrates: 18g; Fiber: 5g; Protein: 2g; Calcium: 34mg; Vitamin D: 0mcg; Vitamin B12: 0mcg; Iron: 2mg; Zinc: 1mg

Coconut-Melon Cooler

Serves 4 / Prep time: 5 mins

DAIRY-FREE   GLUTEN-FREE   NUT-FREE   SOY-FREE

HYPOGLYCEMIA POWER FOOD, LOW-FODMAP FOR IBS, HASHIMOTO'S POWER FOOD, BRAIN FOG, MOOD BOOSTER, FIBROMYALGIA POWER FOOD, TOXIN BUSTER

This is a perfect frozen drink for a hot summer day, when super-sweet melons are at their peak. This recipe calls for cantaloupe, but it also works well with honeydew. This is a great drink to make ahead a few hours before friends come over and keep chilled in the refrigerator until they arrive. This recipe can also be frozen in a mold to make fruit popsicles.

4 cups fresh cantaloupe, peeled and diced

1 cup coconut water

½ cup ice

2 tablespoons freshly squeezed lime juice

5 fresh mint leaves (optional)

In a blender, combine the cantaloupe, coconut water, ice, lime juice, and mint leaves (if using). Blend for 30 seconds, or until smooth. Serve immediately.

Substitution Tip: If the melon you're using isn't sweet enough, you can add 1 tablespoon of maple syrup. If you have Hashimoto's, **Fibromyalgia**, or **Toxin Overload**, avoid maple syrup and instead use one or two pitted medjool dates.

Per serving: Calories: 73; Total fat: 0g; Carbohydrates: 17g; Fiber: 2g; Protein: 2g; Calcium: 31mg; Vitamin D: 0mcg; Vitamin B12: 0mcg; Iron: 1mg; Zinc: 0mg

Chocolate-Mint Nice Cream

Serves 6 to 8 / Prep time: 5 mins, plus freezing overnight

DAIRY-FREE   GLUTEN-FREE   NUT-FREE   SOY-FREE

HYPOGLYCEMIA POWER FOOD, BRAIN FOG, MOOD BOOSTER

This delicious homemade chocolate-mint nice cream can be made without an ice cream maker! Bananas serve as the base for this recipe (and provide a natural sweetener), but I also add avocados for extra creaminess. Make this recipe a day ahead so you have time to freeze it overnight. Note: Both components of this recipe use maple syrup, so if you have Hashimoto's disease, try the Strawberry-Banana Nice Cream (page 138) instead.

2 ripe bananas
2 avocados
½ cup canned coconut milk
1 teaspoon mint extract

⅛ cup pure maple syrup
¼ cup Dark Chocolate Dipper sauce
  (page 140)

1. In a blender, combine the bananas, avocados, coconut milk, mint extract, and maple syrup and blend until smooth. Transfer the mixture to an airtight container, drizzle with the Dark Chocolate Dipper sauce, and stir to incorporate.

2. Freeze the container overnight before serving. The nice cream will retain its creamy texture in the freezer for up to 1 week.

Substitution Tip: You can also try using honey as a replacement for maple syrup or using fresh mint leaves instead of or in addition to mint extract.

Per serving: Calories: 248; Total fat: 15g; Carbohydrates: 23g; Fiber: 7g; Protein: 3g; Calcium: 25mg; Vitamin D: 0mcg; Vitamin B12: 0mcg; Iron: 1mg; Zinc: 1mg

Nutty Blueberry Smoothie

Serves 3 / **Prep time: 5 mins**

DAIRY-FREE   GLUTEN-FREE   NUT-FREE   SOY-FREE

HYPOGLYCEMIA POWER FOOD, INSOMNIA, BRAIN FOG, MOOD BOOSTER,
FIBROMYALGIA POWER FOOD, TOXIN BUSTER

So many of my clients start their days with smoothies and smoothie bowls, thinking they're a healthy and nutritious choice. They may well be, but the ingredients make all the difference. If a smoothie is made with only fruits, it will be too high in carbohydrates, leaving you hungry an hour later. A nutritious smoothie should contain low-sugar fruits (like berries), in addition to fiber, fat, and protein to prevent a sugar crash. This recipe uses frozen cauliflower and chia seeds to boost fiber intake.

1 cup frozen blueberries
1 cup frozen cauliflower florets
1 cup unsweetened plant-based milk
1 medjool date, pitted
1 tablespoon chia seeds

Juice of ½ lemon
½ cup ice
Plant-based milk or water, as needed
   for thinning

In a blender, combine the blueberries, cauliflower, milk, date, chia seeds, lemon juice, and ice and blend for 1 to 2 minutes, or until creamy. If the smoothie is too thick, add milk 1 tablespoon at a time to thin to a pourable consistency. Enjoy immediately.

Substitution Tip: You can add an equal amount of flaxseed or hemp seeds instead of or in addition to the chia seeds.

Per serving: Calories: 107; Total fat: 2g; Carbohydrates: 20g; Fiber: 4g; Protein: 4g; Calcium: 104mg; Vitamin D: 8mcg; Vitamin B12: 1mcg; Iron: 1mg; Zinc: 0mg

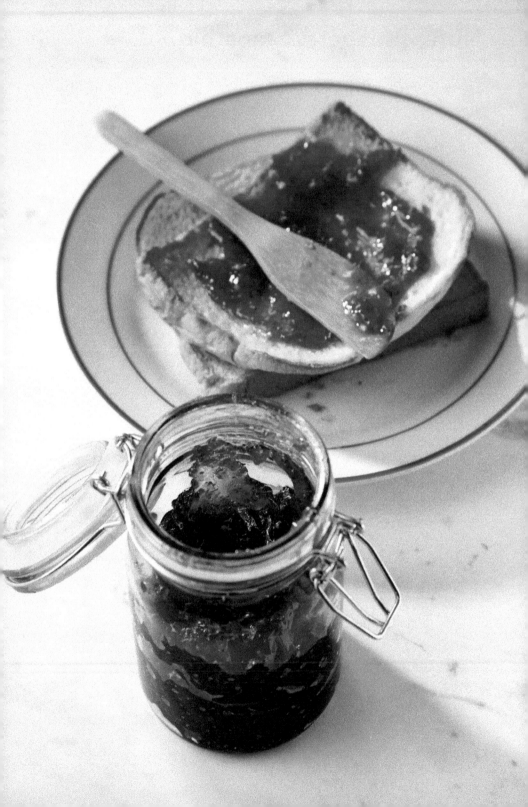

Chapter 11

Basic Staples, Condiments, Dressings, and More

Creamy Tahini Dressing

Makes ½ cup (4 servings) / **Prep time: 5 mins**

DAIRY-FREE   GLUTEN-FREE   NUT-FREE   SOY-FREE

LOW-FODMAP FOR IBS, BRAIN FOG, MOOD BOOSTER, HASHIMOTO'S POWER FOOD, FIBROMYALGIA POWER FOOD, TOXIN BUSTER

Tahini, which is made of ground sesame seeds, serves as the base of this creamy dressing and offers nutrients including B vitamins and anti-oxidants. This dressing pairs nicely with green salads, grain bowls, and roasted vegetables or chicken. Depending on how you're using it, you can add or omit water to adjust the dressing's thickness. Investing in high-quality tahini will bring this dressing up a notch!

2 tablespoons tahini

2 tablespoons freshly squeezed lemon juice

2 tablespoons extra-virgin olive oil

1 garlic clove, grated ◆ / ▣

2 tablespoons water

In a small bowl, combine the tahini, lemon juice, olive oil, garlic, and water. Stir or whisk until the dressing is smooth and creamy but thin enough to drizzle. Refrigerate for up to 1 week.

Substitution Tip: If you have IBS or Fibromyalgia, omit the garlic and use garlic-infused olive oil in place of regular olive oil.

Per serving: Calories: 107; Total fat: 11g; Carbohydrates: 2g; Fiber: 1g; Protein: 1g; Calcium: 34mg; Vitamin D: 0mcg; Vitamin B12: 0mcg; Iron: 1mg; Zinc: 0mg

Peruvian Green Spicy Sauce

Makes 1 cup (16 servings) / **Prep time: 5 mins** / **Cook time: 10 mins**

DAIRY-FREE   GLUTEN-FREE   NUT-FREE   SOY-FREE

INSOMNIA, BRAIN FOG, MOOD BOOSTER, TOXIN BUSTER

This sauce, called *aji verde*, is frequently served as part of a Peruvian-style chicken dish (the chicken is usually rubbed with garlic, oregano, cumin, and paprika and roasted). I have found that *aji verde* is really versatile in the kitchen, so I use it on chicken, grain bowls, salads, fish, and Roasted Summer Vegetables (page 131).

1 jalapeño pepper, seeded
1 serrano pepper, seeded
3 garlic cloves ◆ / ■
2 bunches cilantro, stemmed

¼ cup avocado oil
¼ teaspoon kosher salt
¼ cup water, plus more as needed

In a blender, combine the jalapeño pepper, serrano pepper, garlic, cilantro, avocado oil, salt, and water and blend until creamy. Add about ⅛ cup more water if the sauce is too thick. Store in an airtight container for 2 weeks in the refrigerator.

Substitution Tip: You can replace the avocado oil with olive oil if desired. If you have **IBS** or **Fibromyalgia**, omit the garlic and use garlic-infused avocado oil or olive oil.

Per serving: Calories: 33; Total fat: 3g; Carbohydrates: 1g; Fiber: 0g; Protein: 0g; Calcium: 3mg; Vitamin D: 0mcg; Vitamin B12: 0mcg; Iron: 0mg; Zinc: 0mg

Creamy Vanilla Cashew Milk

Makes 1 quart (4 to 6 servings) / Prep time: 2 mins, plus 4 hours soaking

DAIRY-FREE   GLUTEN-FREE   SOY-FREE

HYPOGLYCEMIA POWER FOOD, INSOMNIA, BRAIN FOG, MOOD BOOSTER, HASHIMOTO'S POWER FOOD, TOXIN BUSTER

I recommend my clients make their own plant-based milk if they can. There are only a few brands I feel comfortable recommending to clients, and even those have their issues. I recommend soaking the cashews (or other nuts) overnight so they're ready to go the next day. Or try the 30-second nut milk method in the Too Tired to Cook tip after the recipe.

4 cups water

1 cup raw unsalted cashews soaked in 3 cups water for at least 4 hours, drained ◆

½ teaspoon ground cinnamon

⅛ teaspoon kosher salt

½ teaspoon alcohol- and sugar-free vanilla extract

¼ teaspoon chopped vanilla bean (optional)

1. In a blender, combine the water, soaked and drained cashews, cinnamon, salt, vanilla, and vanilla bean (if using). Blend for about 2 minutes, or until the mixture is creamy.

2. Store the milk in the refrigerator for up to 2 weeks and shake well before serving. To reheat, microwave 6 ounces for 30 to 40 seconds.

Too Tired to Cook: No time to soak the nuts? Use nut butter instead. Combine 2 tablespoons of nut butter, 2 cups of water, and ½ teaspoon of vanilla extract in a blender, and blend until creamy.

Substitution Tip: If you have IBS or are sensitive to cashews, you can make this recipe with other nuts, like peanuts (recommended for IBS) or blanched almonds.

Per serving: Calories: 50; Total fat: 3g; Carbohydrates: 7g; Fiber: 0g; Protein: 1g; Calcium: 300mg; Vitamin D: 6mcg; Vitamin B12: 1mcg; Iron: 1mg; Zinc: 0mg

Spicy Tomato Salsa

Makes 2 cups (12 servings) / **Prep time: 5 mins** / **Cook time: 10 mins**

DAIRY-FREE GLUTEN-FREE NUT-FREE SOY-FREE

INSOMNIA, BRAIN FOG, MOOD BOOSTER, TOXIN BUSTER

High-quality tomato salsa without preservatives can be difficult to find. Store-bought varieties are usually loaded with sugar, salt, and additives. This salsa uses highly nutritious ingredients and is really easy to make. Serve it with eggs, avocados, or roasted chicken or fish. I also recommend it with Shrimp Tacos with Black Bean Salad (page 121).

3 medium tomatoes, chopped

1 garlic clove, chopped ◆ / ■

1 jalapeño pepper, seeded
  and chopped

1 tablespoon extra-virgin olive oil

¼ onion, finely chopped ◆ / ■

¼ bunch cilantro, finely chopped
  (about ½ cup chopped)

¼ teaspoon kosher salt

1. In a food processor, combine the tomatoes, garlic, and jalapeño and pulse until minced.

2. Heat the olive oil in a large skillet over medium-high heat, add the tomato mixture, and cook for 3 to 5 minutes, or until it begins to boil.

3. Transfer the mixture to a large bowl. Add the onion, cilantro, and salt.

4. Let the salsa cool completely before pouring into an airtight container. Refrigerate for up to 1 week.

Substitution Tip: If you have IBS or Fibromyalgia, omit the garlic and use garlic-infused olive oil, and replace the onion with the green portions of 1 or 2 scallions. If you want spicier salsa, leave the seeds in the jalapeño.

Per serving: Calories: 17; Total fat: 1g; Carbohydrates: 2g; Fiber: 1g; Protein: 0g; Calcium: 5mg; Vitamin D: 0mcg; Vitamin B12: 0mcg; Iron: 0mg; Zinc: 0mg

Quick Pickled Red Onions

Makes 2 cups (8 to 12 servings) / **Prep time: 5 mins, plus 30 mins pickling time**

DAIRY-FREE   GLUTEN-FREE   NUT-FREE   SOY-FREE

INSOMNIA, BRAIN FOG, MOOD BOOSTER, HASHIMOTO'S POWER FOOD, LOW-FODMAP FOR IBS, TOXIN BUSTER

Pickling is usually a slow process that involves making a brine and then marinating vegetables long-term, often for months. Luckily, this quick-pickling method takes just 30 minutes and offers an acidic burst of flavor to balance any of the savory dishes in this book. Personally, I love these onions with Hearty Black Bean Burgers (page 86) and Shakshuka (page 80).

1 or 2 red onions, thinly sliced ◆ / ■   1½ cups Champagne vinegar

Put the sliced onions in a large jar and pour in the Champagne vinegar. Use a spoon or spatula to pack the onions down, ensuring they are submerged in the vinegar. Let the mixture sit at room temperature for 30 minutes to 1 hour before serving. Refrigerate for 3 to 4 weeks.

Substitution Tip: If you have IBS or Fibromyalgia, try using thinly sliced radishes instead of onions. I use Champagne vinegar because it is milder in flavor and acidity than apple cider vinegar. If you only have access to apple cider vinegar, use ½ cup of vinegar and 1 cup of water, and add 2 tablespoons of maple syrup. (If you have Hashimoto's, **Fibromyalgia**, or **Toxin Overload**, omit the maple syrup.)

Per serving (2 cups): Calories: 13; Total fat: 0g; Carbohydrates: 3g; Fiber: 1g; Protein: 0g; Calcium: 7mg; Vitamin D: 0mcg; Vitamin B12: 0mcg; Iron: 0mg; Zinc: 0mg

Dijon Mustard Vinaigrette

Makes ½ cup (4 servings) / **Prep time: 5 mins**

DAIRY-FREE   GLUTEN-FREE   NUT-FREE   SOY-FREE

INSOMNIA, BRAIN FOG, MOOD BOOSTER, LOW-FODMAP FOR IBS, HASHIMOTO'S POWER FOOD, FIBROMYALGIA POWER FOOD, TOXIN BUSTER

This is my go-to salad dressing all year round. I usually use upcycled mason jars to make this dressing—simply put the ingredients in the jar and shake it. Use this dressing on roasted vegetables or salads, like the Quinoa and Arugula Salad with Vegetables (page 82), Crunchy Summer Salad (page 85), or Simple Base Salad (page 133). This dressing is still delicious without shallots, though they do add a lot of flavor.

⅓ cup extra-virgin olive oil
2 tablespoons sherry vinegar
½ tablespoon Dijon mustard

⅛ tablespoon kosher salt
1 tablespoon minced shallots ◆ / ■
(optional)

In a small jar with a lid, combine the olive oil, sherry vinegar, Dijon mustard, salt, and shallots (if using). Close the jar and shake well until combined. Refrigerate for up to 2 weeks and shake to combine before serving.

Substitution Tip: If you have IBS or Fibromyalgia, omit the shallots. If you don't have sherry vinegar, you can use red-wine vinegar, or 1½ tablespoons of freshly squeezed lemon juice plus ¼ tablespoon of lemon zest.

Per serving: Calories: 160; Total fat: 18g; Carbohydrates: 0g; Fiber: 0g; Protein: 0g; Calcium: 2mg; Vitamin D: 0mcg; Vitamin B12: 0mcg; Iron: 0mg; Zinc: 0mg

Red Berry Jam

Makes 3 cups (8 to 12 servings) / Prep time: 5 mins / Cook time: 25 mins

DAIRY-FREE   GLUTEN-FREE   NUT-FREE   SOY-FREE

HYPOGLYCEMIA POWER FOOD, INSOMNIA, BRAIN FOG, MOOD BOOSTER, HASHIMOTO'S POWER FOOD, TOXIN BUSTER

I started making this jam-like fruit compote for my son to enjoy at breakfast. It's packed with fiber and vitamins and has no added sugar, and the chia seeds give it a jammy consistency. It's delicious made with in-season berries during the summer or with frozen berries during the winter. Try it on Creamy Chocolate Oatmeal (page 74) or Fluffiest Raspberry Pancakes (page 72), or swirled into plain coconut yogurt with Connor's "Cereal" Granola (page 71).

2 cups fresh or frozen raspberries
2 cups fresh or frozen blueberries
Zest of 1 lemon (about 1 tablespoon)

Juice of ½ lemon (about 1 tablespoon)
¼ cup chia seeds

1. In a medium saucepan, combine the raspberries, blueberries, lemon zest, and lemon juice. Cook over medium heat for about 15 minutes, stirring occasionally with a wooden spoon or spatula to help the fruits break down.

2. Add the chia seeds and stir to incorporate. Cook the mixture for 10 minutes, stirring occasionally and scraping the bottom of the pan to remove stuck bits. The mixture should bubble gently, but if it starts to reach a rolling boil, lower the heat to stop the boiling. Once the mixture is thickened, remove from the heat.

3. Let the jam cool completely before transferring to airtight jars. Refrigerate for 2 to 3 weeks.

Substitution Tip: When fresh berries are not in season, use frozen berries— they are just as nutritious as they are when bought fresh during peak season. You can also add grated fresh ginger for a spicy flavor, depending on your preference.

Per serving: Calories: 48; Total fat: 2g; Carbohydrates: 8g; Fiber: 4g; Protein: 1g; Calcium: 37mg; Vitamin D: 0mcg; Vitamin B12: 0mcg; Iron: 1mg; Zinc: 0mg

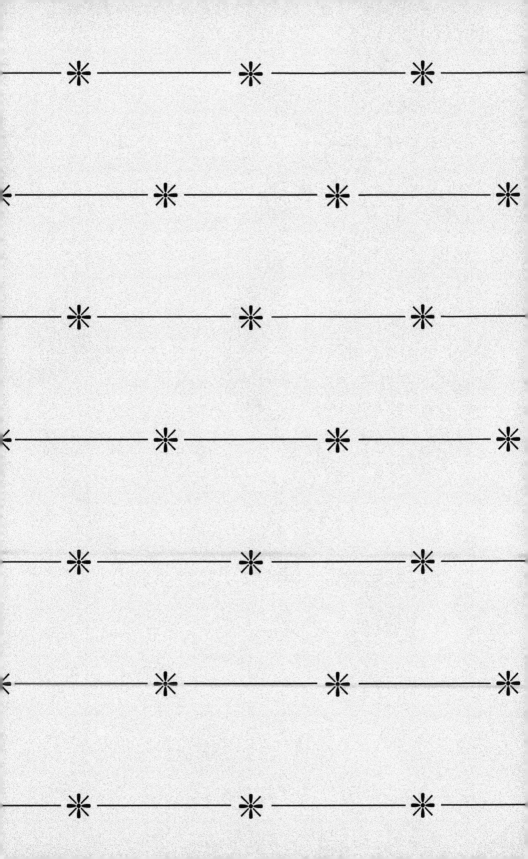

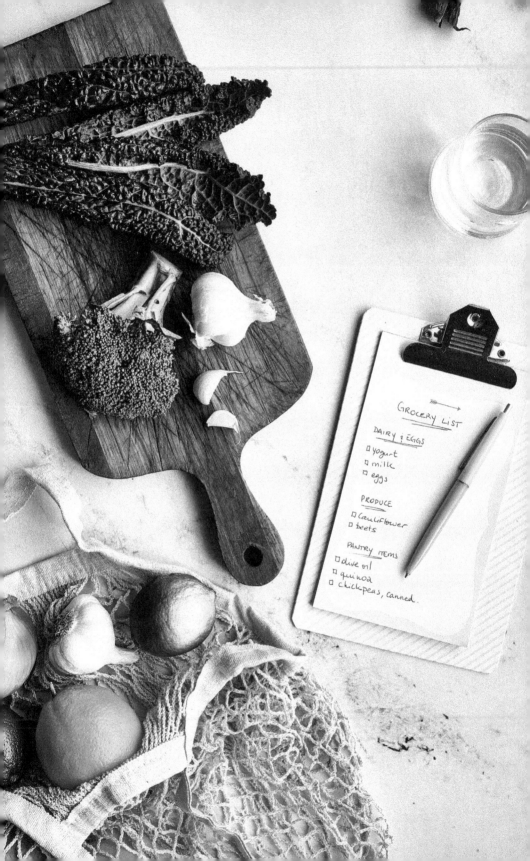

GROCERY LIST

DAIRY & EGGS
☐ yogurt
☐ milk
☐ eggs

PRODUCE
☐ cauliflower
☐ beets

PANTRY ITEMS
☐ olive oil
☐ quinoa
☐ chickpeas, canned

Measurement Conversions

OVEN TEMPERATURES

Fahrenheit (F)	Celsius (C) (approximate)
250°F	120°C
300°F	150°C
325°F	165°C
350°F	180°C
375°F	190°C
400°F	200°C
425°F	220°C
450°F	230°C

WEIGHT EQUIVALENTS

US Standard	Metric (approximate)
½ ounce	15 g
1 ounce	30 g
2 ounces	60 g
4 ounces	115 g
8 ounces	225 g
12 ounces	340 g
16 ounces or 1 pound	455 g

VOLUME EQUIVALENTS (LIQUID)

US Standard	US Standard (ounces)	Metric (approximate)
2 tablespoons	1 fl. oz.	30 mL
¼ cup	2 fl. oz.	60 mL
½ cup	4 fl. oz.	120 mL
1 cup	8 fl. oz.	240 mL
1½ cups	12 fl. oz.	355 mL
2 cups or 1 pint	16 fl. oz.	475 mL
4 cups or 1 quart	32 fl. oz.	1 L
1 gallon	128 fl. oz.	4 L

References

Acheson, Kevin J., Gérard Gremaud, Isabelle Meirim, Franck Montigon, Yves Krebs, Laurent B. Fay, Louis-Jean Gay, Philippe Schneiter, Charles Schindler, and Luc Tappy. "Metabolic Effects of Caffeine in Humans: Lipid Oxidation or Futile Cycling?" *The American Journal of Clinical Nutrition* 79, no. 1 (January 2004): 40–46. doi.org/10.1093/ajcn/79.1.40.

American College of Rheumatology. "What Is a Rheumatologist?" Accessed March 2, 2020. rheumatology.org/I-Am-A/Patient-Caregiver/Health-Care-Team/What-is -a-Rheumatologist.

American Thyroid Association. "Hashimoto's Thyroiditis (Lymphocytic Thyroiditis)." Accessed March 8, 2020. thyroid.org/hashimotos-thyroiditis.

Anglin, Rebecca E. S., Zainab Samaan, Stephen D. Walter, and Sarah D. McDonald. "Vitamin D Deficiency and Depression in Adults: Systematic Review and Meta-Analysis." *The British Journal of Psychiatry* 202, no. 2 (February 2013): 100–107. doi.org /10.1192/bjp.bp.111.106666.

Aronson, Dina. "Cortisol: Its Role in Stress, Inflammation, and Indications for Diet Therapy." *Today's Dietitian* 11, no. 11 (November 2009): 38. TodaysDietitian.com/newarchives /111609p38.shtml.

Bouzari, Ali, Dirk Holstege, and Diane M. Barrett. "Mineral, Fiber, and Total Phenolic Retention in Eight Fruits and Vegetables: A Comparison of Refrigerated and Frozen Storage." *Journal of Agricultural and Food Chemistry* 63, no. 3 (January 28, 2015): 951–56. doi.org/10.1021/jf504890k.

Brown, Amy C, and Ana Valiere. "Probiotics and Medical Nutrition Therapy." *Nutrition in Clinical Care* 7, no. 2 (April–June 2004): 56–68. NCBI.NLM.NIH.gov/pmc/articles /PMC1482314.

Buyken, Annette E., Victoria Flood, Marianne Empson, Elena Rochtchina, Alan W. Barclay, Jennie Brand-Miller, and Paul Mitchell. "Carbohydrate Nutrition and Inflammatory Disease Mortality in Older Adults." *The American Journal of Clinical Nutrition* 92, no. 3 (September 2010): 634–43. doi.org/10.3945/ajcn.2010.29390.

Campbell, Donald. "Hormonal Chaos: The Scientific and Social Origin of the Environmental Endocrine Hypothesis." *British Medical Journal* 321, no. 7259 (August 19, 2000): 516. BMJ.com/content/321/7259/516.2.

Connor, Ann Marie, James J. Luby, James F. Hancock, Steven Berkheimer, and Eric J. Hanson. "Changes in Fruit Antioxidant Activity among Blueberry Cultivars during Cold-Temperature Storage." *Journal of Agricultural and Food Chemistry* 50, no. 4 (February 1, 2002): 893–98. doi.org/10.1021/jf011212y.

Desimone, Marisa E., and Ruth S. Weinstock. "Non-Diabetic Hypoglycemia." In *Endotext* [internet], ed. Kenneth R. Feingold. South Dartmouth, MA: MDText.com, 2000–. September 23, 2017. NCBI.NLM.NIH.gov/books/NBK355894.

DiNicolantonio, James J., James H. O'Keefe, and William L. Wilson. "Sugar Addiction: Is It Real? A Narrative Review." *British Journal of Sports Medicine* 52, no. 14 (July 2018): 910–13. doi.org/10.1136/bjsports-2017-097971.

Djokic, Gorica, Petar Vojvodic, Davor Korcok, Anita Agic, Anica Rankovic, Vladan Djordjevic, Aleksandra Vojvodic, et al. "The Effects of Magnesium–Melatonin–Vit B Complex Supplementation in Treatment of Insomnia." *Open Access Macedonian Journal of Medical* Sciences 7, no. 18 (September 30, 2019): 3101–5. doi.org/10.3889 /oamjms.2019.771.

Dulloo, A. G., C. A. Geissler, T. Horton, A. Collins, and D. S. Miller. "Normal Caffeine Consumption: Influence on Thermogenesis and Daily Energy Expenditure in Lean and Postobese Human Volunteers." *The American Journal of Clinical Nutrition* 49, no. 1 (January 1989): 44–50. doi.org/10.1093/ajcn/49.1.44.

Frazier, Thomas H., John K. DiBaise, and Craig J. McClain. "Gut Microbiota, Intestinal Permeability, Obesity-Induced Inflammation, and Liver Injury." *Journal of Parenteral and Enteral Nutrition* 35, no. 5S (September 2011): 14S–20S. doi.org/10.1177 /0148607111413772.

Fries, Eva, Judith Hesse, Juliane Hellhammer, and Dirk H. Hellhammer. "A New View on Hypocortisolism." *Psychoneuroendocrinology* 30, no. 10 (November 2005): 1010–16. doi.org/10.1016/j.psyneuen.2005.04.006.

Fu, Xin, Betty S. Blaydes, Constance C. Weis, John R. Latendresse, Levan Muskhelishvili, Thomas R. Sutter, and K. Barry Delclos. "Effects of Dietary Soy and Estrous Cycle on Adrenal Cytochrome P450 1B1 Expression and DMBA Metabolism in Adrenal Glands and Livers in Female Sprague-Dawley Rats." *Chemico-Biological Interactions* 146, no. 3 (December 15, 2003): 273–84. doi.org/10.1016/j.cbi.2003.09.004.

Ganmaa, Davaasambuu, and Akio Sato. "The Possible Role of Female Sex Hormones in Milk from Pregnant Cows in the Development of Breast, Ovarian and Corpus Uteri Cancers." *Medical Hypotheses* 65, no. 6 (2005): 1028–37. doi.org/10.1016 /j.mehy.2005.06.026.

Hardy, Rowan, and Mark S. Cooper. "Adrenal Gland and Bone." *Archives of Biochemistry and Biophysics* 503, no. 1 (November 1, 2010): 137–45. doi.org/10.1016/j.abb.2010.06.007.

Harris, Cheryl. "Thyroid Disease and Diet—Nutrition Plays a Part in Maintaining Thyroid Health." *Today's Dietitian* 14, no. 7 (July 2012): 40. TodaysDietitian.com/newarchives /070112p40.shtml.

Heim, Christine, Ulrike Ehlert, and Dirk H. Hellhammer. "The Potential Role of Hypocortisolism in the Pathophysiology of Stress-Related Bodily Disorders." *Psychoneuroendocrinology* 25, no. 1 (January 2000): 1–35. doi.org/10.1016 /s0306-4530(99)00035-9.

Hirotsu, Camila, Sergio Tufik, and Monica Levy Andersen. "Interactions between Sleep, Stress, and Metabolism: From Physiological to Pathological Conditions." *Sleep Science* 8, no. 3 (November 2015): 143–52. doi.org/10.1016/j.slsci.2015.09.002.

Högberg, Göran, Sven A. Gustafsson, Tore Hällström, Tove Gustafsson, Björn Klawitter, and Maria Petersson. "Depressed Adolescents in a Case-Series Were Low in Vitamin D and Depression Was Ameliorated by Vitamin D Supplementation." *Acta Paediatrica* (Oslo, Norway) 101, no. 7 (July 2012): 779–83. doi.org/10.1111/j.1651-2227.2012.02655.x.

Hughes, David A. "Effects of Dietary Antioxidants on the Immune Function of Middle-Aged Adults." *Proceedings of the Nutrition Society* 58, no. 1 (February 1999): 79–84. doi.org/10.1079/pns19990012.

Hyman, Mark. "Systems Biology, Toxins, Obesity, and Functional Medicine." *Alternative Therapies In Health And Medicine* 13, no. 2 (March–April 2007): S134–39.

Jahnen-Dechent, Wilhelm, and Markus Ketteler. "Magnesium Basics." *Clinical Kidney Journal* 5, supplement 1 (February 1, 2012): i3–i14. doi.org/10.1093/ndtplus/sfr163.

Johns Hopkins Medicine. "The Brain-Gut Connection." Accessed April 5, 2020. HopkinsMedicine.org/health/wellness-and-prevention/the-brain-gut-connection.

Kiecolt-Glaser, Janice K., Heather M. Derry, and Christopher P. Fagundes. "Inflammation: Depression Fans the Flames and Feasts on the Heat." *American Journal of Psychiatry* 172, no. 11 (November 1, 2015): 1075–91. doi.org/10.1176/appi.ajp.2015.15020152.

Koot, Paula, and Paul Deurenberg. "Comparison of Changes in Energy Expenditure and Body Temperatures after Caffeine Consumption." *Annals of Nutrition and Metabolism* 39, no. 3 (1995): 135–42. doi.org/10.1159/000177854.

Krimsky, Sheldon. *Hormonal Chaos: The Scientific and Social Origins of the Environmental Endocrine Hypothesis*. Baltimore: Johns Hopkins University Press, 2000.

Krysiak, Robert, Witold Szkróbka, and Bogusław Okopień. "The Effect of Gluten-Free Diet on Thyroid Autoimmunity in Drug-Naïve Women with Hashimoto's Thyroiditis: A Pilot Study." *Experimental and Clinical Endocrinology and Diabetes* 127, no. 7 (July 2019): 417–22. doi.org/10.1055/a-0653-7108.

Mayo Clinic. "Primary Immunodeficiency." January 30, 2020. MayoClinic.org/diseases-conditions/primary-immunodeficiency/symptoms-causes/syc-20376905.

Meletis, Chris D., and Wayne A. Centrone. "Adrenal Fatigue: Enhancing Quality of Life for Patients with a Functional Disorder." *Alternative and Complementary Therapies* 8, no. 5 (October 2002): 267–72. doi.org/10.1089/107628002760396418.

Montonen, Jukka, Heiner Boeing, Andreas Fritsche, Erwin Schleicher, Hans-Georg Joost, Matthias B. Schulze, Annika Steffen, and Tobias Pischon. "Consumption of Red Meat and Whole-Grain Bread in Relation to Biomarkers of Obesity, Inflammation, Glucose Metabolism and Oxidative Stress." *European Journal of Nutrition* 52, no. 1 (February 2013): 337–45. doi.org/10.1007/s00394-012-0340-6.

Moriguchi, Satoru, and Mikako Muraga. "Vitamin E and Immunity." *Vitamins and Hormones* 59 (2000): 305–36. doi.org/10.1016/s0083-6729(00)59011-6.

Munro, Malcolm G., Hilary O. D. Critchley, and Ian S. Fraser. "The FIGO Systems for Nomenclature and Classification of Causes of Abnormal Uterine Bleeding in the Reproductive Years: Who Needs Them?" *American Journal of Obstetrics and Gynecology* 207, no. 4 (October 1, 2012): 259–65. doi.org/10.1016/j.ajog .2012.01.046.

National Institutes of Health, Eunice Kennedy Shriver National Institute of Child Health and Human Development. "What Are the Common Treatments for Menstrual Irregularities?" January 31, 2017. NICHD.NIH.gov/health/topics/menstruation /conditioninfo/treatments.

National Institutes of Health, Eunice Kennedy Shriver National Institute of Child Health and Human Development. "What Causes Menstrual Irregularities?" January 31, 2017. NICHD.NIH.gov/health/topics/menstruation/conditioninfo/causes.

National Institutes of Health, National Center for Complementary and Integrative Health. "Fibromyalgia: In Depth." March 27, 2018. NCCIH.NIH.gov/health/fibromyalgia-in-depth.

National Institutes of Health, National Institute of Diabetes and Digestive and Kidney Diseases. "Irritable Bowel Syndrome (IBS)." Accessed March 2, 2020. NIDDK.NIH.gov /health-information/digestive-diseases/irritable-bowel-syndrome.

National Institutes of Health, National Institute of Diabetes and Digestive and Kidney Diseases."Treatment for Adrenal Insufficiency and Addison's Disease." September 1, 2018. NIDDK.NIH.gov/health-information/endocrine-diseases/adrenal-insufficiency -addisons-disease/treatment.

National Institutes of Health, National Institute of Mental Health. "5 Things You Should Know About Stress." Accessed March 2, 2020. NIMH.NIH.gov/health/publications /stress/index.shtml.

National Institutes of Health, National Institute of Mental Health. "Depression." Accessed March 8, 2020. NIMH.NIH.gov/health/topics/depression/index.shtml.

National Osteoporosis Foundation. "Bone Density Exam/Testing." Accessed March 10, 2020. NOF.org/patients/diagnosis-information/bone-density-examtesting.

Ocon, Anthony J. "Caught in the Thickness of Brain Fog: Exploring the Cognitive Symptoms of Chronic Fatigue Syndrome." *Frontiers in Physiology* 4 (April 2013): 63. doi.org/10.3389/fphys.2013.00063.

Page, Kathleen A., Dongju Seo, Renata Belfort-DeAguiar, Cheryl Lacadie, James Dzuira, Sarita Naik, Suma Amarnath, R. Todd Constable, Robert S. Sherwin, and Rajita Sinha. "Circulating Glucose Levels Modulate Neural Control of Desire for High-Calorie Foods in Humans." *Journal of Clinical Investigation* 121, no. 10 (October 3, 2011): 4161–69. doi.org/10.1172/jci57873.

Palmer, Sharon. "Is There a Link between Nutrition and Autoimmune Disease?" *Today's Dietitian* 13, no. 11 (November 2011): 36. TodaysDietitian.com/newarchives /110211p36.shtml.

Parekh, Ranna. "What Is Depression?" American Psychiatric Association. January 2017. psychiatry.org/patients-families/depression/what-is-depression.

Qin, Hong-Yan, Chung-Wah Cheng, Xu-Dong Tang, and Zhao-Xiang Bian. "Impact of Psychological Stress on Irritable Bowel Syndrome." *World Journal of Gastroenterology* 20, no. 39 (October 21, 2014): 14126–31. doi.org/10.3748/wjg.v20.i39.14126.

Quirk, Shae E., Lana J. Williams, Adrienne O'Neil, Julie A. Pasco, Felice N. Jacka, Siobhan Housden, Michael Berk, and Sharon L. Brennan. "The Association between Diet Quality, Dietary Patterns and Depression in Adults: A Systematic Review." *BMC Psychiatry* 13 (June 27, 2013): 175. doi.org/10.1186/1471-244x-13-175.

Rachdaoui, Nadia, and Dipak K. Sarkar. "Effects of Alcohol on the Endocrine System." *Endocrinology and Metabolism Clinics of North America* 42, no. 3 (September 2013): 593–615. doi.org/10.1016/j.ecl.2013.05.008.

Reid, Gregor, Jana Jass, M. Tom Sebulsky, and John K. McCormick. "Potential Uses of Probiotics in Clinical Practice." *Clinical Microbiology Reviews* 16, no. 4 (October 2003): 658–72. doi.org/10.1128/cmr.16.4.658-672.2003.

Resta-Lenert, S., and K. E. Barrett. "Live Probiotics Protect Intestinal Epithelial Cells from the Effects of Infection with Enteroinvasive *Escherichia coli* (EIEC)." *Gut* 52, no. 7 (July 2003): 988–97. doi.org/10.1136/gut.52.7.988.

Romm, Aviva. "Adrenal Fatigue Syndrome: Integrative Treatment Approach for an Evolving Diagnosis." *Alternative and Complementary Therapies* 21, no. 6 (December 21, 2015): 242–46. doi.org/10.1089/act.2015.29028.aro.

Sarris, Jerome, Alan C. Logan, Tasnime N. Akbaraly, G. Paul Amminger, Vicent Balanzá-Martínez, Marlene P. Freeman, Joseph Hibbeln, et al. "Nutritional Medicine as Mainstream in Psychiatry." *The Lancet Psychiatry* 2, no. 3 (March 1, 2015): 271–74. doi.org/10.1016/s2215-0366(14)00051-0.

Sathyapalan, Thozhukat, Alireza M. Manuchehri, Natalie J. Thatcher, Alan S. Rigby, Tom Chapman, Eric S. Kilpatrick, and Stephen L. Atkin. "The Effect of Soy Phytoestrogen Supplementation on Thyroid Status and Cardiovascular Risk Markers in Patients with Subclinical Hypothyroidism: A Randomized, Double-Blind, Crossover Study." *Journal of Clinical Endocrinology and Metabolism* 96, no. 5 (May 1, 2011): 1442–49. doi.org/10.1210/jc.2010-2255.

Silbergeld, Ellen K., Jay Graham, and Lance B. Price. "Industrial Food Animal Production, Antimicrobial Resistance, and Human Health." *Annual Review of Public Health* 29 (2008): 151–69. doi.org/10.1146/annurev.publhealth.29.020907.090904.

Smeets, Paul A. M., Cees de Graaf, Annette Stafleu, Matthias J. P. van Osch, and Jeroen van der Grond. "Functional Magnetic Resonance Imaging of Human Hypothalamic Responses to Sweet Taste and Calories." *The American Journal of Clinical Nutrition* 82, no. 5 (November 2005): 1011–16. doi.org/10.1093/ajcn/82.5.1011.

Sørensen, Lone B., Anne Raben, Steen Stender, and Arne Astrup. "Effect of Sucrose on Inflammatory Markers in Overweight Humans." *The American Journal of Clinical Nutrition* 82, no. 2 (August 2005): 421–27. doi.org/https://doi.org/10.1093/ajcn/82.2.421.

Spiegel, Brennan M. R., Mary Farid, Eric Esrailian, Jennifer Talley, and Lin Chang. "Is Irritable Bowel Syndrome a Diagnosis of Exclusion? A Survey of Primary Care Providers, Gastroenterologists, and IBS Experts." *American Journal of Gastroenterology* 105, no. 4 (April 2010): 848–58. doi.org/10.1038/ajg.2010.47.

Spreadbury, Ian. "Comparison with Ancestral Diets Suggests Dense Acellular Carbohydrates Promote an Inflammatory Microbiota, and May Be the Primary Dietary Cause of Leptin Resistance and Obesity." *Diabetes, Metabolic Syndrome and Obesity: Targets and Therapy* 5 (2012): 175–89. doi.org/10.2147/DMSO.S33473.

Stedman, Thomas Lathrop. *Stedman's Medical Dictionary*. 28th ed. Philadelphia: Lippincott Williams & Wilkins, 2006.

Steinfeld, Henning, Pierre Gerber, Tom Wassenaar, Vincent Castel, Mauricio Rosales, and Cees de Haan. "Livestock's Long Shadow: Environmental Issues and Options." United Nations, Food and Agriculture Organization. 2006. FAO.org/3/a0701e/a0701e00.pdf.

Stewart, E. A. "Irritable Bowel Syndrome—An Overview of Treatment Options." *Today's Dietitian* 16, no. 4 (April 2014): 46. TodaysDietitian.com/newarchives/040114p46.shtml.

Strieder, Thea G. A., Mark F. Prummel, Jan G. P. Tijssen, Eric Endert, and Wilmar M. Wiersinga. "Risk Factors for and Prevalence of Thyroid Disorders in a Cross-Sectional Study among Healthy Female Relatives of Patients with Autoimmune Thyroid Disease." *Clinical Endocrinology* 59, no. 3 (September 2003): 396–401. doi.org/10.1046/j.1365-2265.2003.01862.x.

Takeda, Eiji, Junji Terao, Yutaka Nakaya, Ken-ichi Miyamoto, Yoshinobu Baba, Hiroshi Chuman, Ryuji Kaji, Tetsuro Ohmori, and Kazuhito Rokutan. "Stress Control and Human Nutrition." *Journal of Medical Investigation* 51, no. 3–4 (August 2004): 139–45. doi.org/10.2152/jmi.51.139.

Tomas, Cara, Julia Newton, and Stuart Watson. "A Review of Hypothalamic-Pituitary-Adrenal Axis Function in Chronic Fatigue Syndrome." *ISRN Neuroscience* 2013 (September 30, 2013): 784520. doi.org/10.1155/2013/784520.

Tučková, Ludmila, Helena Tlaskalová-Hogenová, Maria A. Farré, Kamila Karská, Pavel Rossmann, Jiřina Kolínská, and Petr Kocna. "Molecular Mimicry as a Possible Cause of Autoimmune Reactions in Celiac Disease? Antibodies to Gliadin Cross-React with Epitopes on Enterocytes." *Clinical Immunology and Immunopathology* 74, no. 2 (February 1995): 170–76. doi.org/10.1006/clin.1995.1025.

U.S. Food and Drug Administration. "Spilling the Beans: How Much Caffeine Is Too Much?" December 12, 2018. FDA.gov/consumers/consumer-updates/spilling-beans-how-much-caffeine-too-much.

Uygun, David S., Zhiwen Ye, Anna Y. Zecharia, Edward C. Harding, Xiao Yu, Raquel Yustos, Alexei L. Vyssotski, Stephen G. Brickley, Nicholas P. Franks, and William Wisden. "Bottom-Up versus Top-Down Induction of Sleep by Zolpidem Acting on Histaminergic and Neocortex Neurons." *Journal of Neuroscience* 36, no. 44 (November 2, 2016): 11171–84. doi.org/10.1523/jneurosci.3714-15.2016.

Victoria, Australia, Department of Health and Human Services. "Fatigue." June 30, 2015. BetterHealth.vic.gov.au/health/conditionsandtreatments/fatigue.

Vighi, G., F. Marcucci, L. Sensi, G. Di Cara, and F. Frati. "Allergy and the Gastrointestinal System." *Clinical and Experimental Immunology* 153, no. S1 (September 2008): 3–6. doi.org/10.1111/j.1365-2249.2008.03713.x.

Wilson, James L. "Clinical Perspective on Stress, Cortisol and Adrenal Fatigue." *Advances in Integrative Medicine* 1, no. 2 (May 2014): 93–96. doi.org/10.1016/j.aimed.2014.05.002.

Wright, K. C. "Clinical Nutrition: Beyond Food and Mood." *Today's Dietitian* 21, no. 7 (July 2019): 10. TodaysDietitian.com/newarchives/0719p10.shtml.

Yancey, Joseph R., and Sarah M. Thomas. "Chronic Fatigue Syndrome: Diagnosis and Treatment." *American Family Physician* 86, no. 8 (October 15, 2012): 741–46. aafp.org/afp/2012/1015/p741.html.

Yang, Qing. "Gain Weight by 'Going Diet?' Artificial Sweeteners and the Neurobiology of Sugar Cravings: Neuroscience 2010." *Yale Journal of Biology and Medicine* 83, no. 2 (June 2010): 101–8. NCBI.NLM.NIH.gov/pmc/articles/PMC2892765.

Resources

American College of Rheumatology (for fibromyalgia):
rheumatology.org

American Diabetes Association (ADA) (for hypoglycemia):
diabetes.org

American Lung Association (for straw breathing technique):
Lung.org (search "pursed lip breathing" for video)

American Thyroid Association:
thyroid.org

Anxiety and Depression Association of America (for depression and anxiety):
ADAA.org

Center for Mindful Eating:
TheCenterforMindfulEating.org

Environmental Working Group (EWG) (for toxin overload):
EWG.org

FODY Foods (for IBS food products):
FodyFoods.com

Monash University FODMAP diet app (for IBS):
MonashFODMAP.com

National Alliance on Mental Illness (for depression):
nami.org

National Institutes of Health:
NIH.gov

National Sleep Foundation (for insomnia):
SleepFoundation.org

Substance Abuse and Mental Health Services Administration (SAMHSA) (for depression):
SAMHSA.gov

Recipe Index by Symptom

I

Insomnia

Apple-Chia Power Muffins, 69–70
Baked Mustard Salmon, 116
Best Turkey Burgers, 117
Butternut Squash Nest Eggs, 68
Chicken Bone Broth, 106–107
Chicken Tikka Masala Grain Bowl, 94–95
Connor's "Cereal" Granola, 71
Connor's Chicken Soup, 104–105
Creamy Chocolate Oatmeal, 74
Creamy Masoor Dal Grain Bowl, 92–93
Creamy Vanilla Cashew Milk, 148
Crispy Chicken Tenders, 123–124
Crispy Falafel Bowl, 98–99
Crunchy Summer Salad, 85
Dijon Mustard Vinaigrette, 151
Flourless Chickpea Blondies, 139
Fluffiest Raspberry Pancakes, 72–73
Hearty Black Bean Burgers, 86–87
Kabocha Squash Soup, 108
Lazy Day Italian Wedding Soup, 109
Lentil-Spinach Fritters, 81
Muffin Tin Frittatas, 76–77
Nutty Blueberry Smoothie, 143
One-Pot Chicken and Quinoa, 83–84
Peruvian Green Spicy Sauce, 147
Quick Pickled Red Onions, 150
Quinoa and Arugula Salad
    with Vegetables, 82
Red Berry Jam, 152
Roasted Eggplant Ragù, 119–120
Roasted Vegetable Chili, 110–111
Roasted Vegetable Fried Rice, 96–97
Roasted Vegetable Grain Bowl, 90–91
Sautéed Broccoli with Raisins, 130
Sautéed Mushroom and
    Quinoa Bowl, 100
Shakshuka, 80
Shrimp Tacos with Black
    Bean Salad, 121–122
Spicy Tomato Salsa, 149

30-Minute Chicken Pho, 112–113
Uplift Green Smoothie, 75
Warm Green Lentil Salad, 118

L

Low-FODMAP for IBS

Apple-Chia Power Muffins, 69–70
Baked Mustard Salmon, 116
Best Turkey Burgers, 117
Butternut Squash Nest Eggs, 68
Cashew Butter Cups, 137
Chocolate Energy Bites, 136
Cilantro-Lime Rice, 128
Coconut-Melon Cooler, 141
Connor's "Cereal" Granola, 71
Creamy Chocolate Oatmeal, 74
Creamy Tahini Dressing, 146
Dark Chocolate Dipper, 140
Dijon Mustard Vinaigrette, 151
Flourless Chickpea Blondies, 139
Fluffiest Raspberry Pancakes, 72–73
Kabocha Squash Soup, 108
Lazy Day Italian Wedding Soup, 109
Lentil-Spinach Fritters, 81
Quick Pickled Red Onions, 150
Quinoa and Arugula Salad
    with Vegetables, 82
Roasted Sweet Potato "Hummus," 129
Sautéed Broccoli with Raisins, 130
Shakshuka, 80
Simple Base Salad, 133
Uplift Green Smoothie, 75
Warm Green Lentil Salad, 118

M

Mood boosters

Apple-Chia Power Muffins, 69–70
Baked Mustard Salmon, 116
Best Turkey Burgers, 117
Butternut Squash Nest Eggs, 68
Cashew Butter Cups, 137

T

Toxin busters

Ingredient Index

Chia seeds (*continued*)
Creamy Chocolate Oatmeal, 74
Nutty Blueberry Smoothie, 143
Red Berry Jam, 152
Uplift Green Smoothie, 75

Chicken
Chicken Bone Broth, 106–107
Chicken Tikka Masala Grain Bowl, 94–95
Connor's Chicken Soup, 104–105
Crispy Chicken Tenders, 123–124
One-Pot Chicken and Quinoa, 83–84
30-Minute Chicken Pho, 112–113

Chickpeas
Crispy Falafel Bowl, 98–99
Flourless Chickpea Blondies, 139
Quinoa and Arugula Salad
with Vegetables, 82
Shakshuka, 80

Chocolate
Cashew Butter Cups, 137
Chocolate Energy Bites, 136
Chocolate-Mint Nice Cream, 142
Creamy Chocolate Oatmeal, 74
Dark Chocolate Dipper, 140

Cilantro
Best Turkey Burgers, 117
Cilantro-Lime Rice, 128
Hearty Black Bean Burgers, 86–87
Lentil-Spinach Fritters, 81
Peruvian Green Spicy Sauce, 147
Shrimp Tacos with Black
Bean Salad, 121–122
Spicy Tomato Salsa, 149
30-Minute Chicken Pho, 112–113
Warm Green Lentil Salad, 118

Coconut milk
Chocolate-Mint Nice Cream, 142

Coconut water
Coconut-Melon Cooler, 141
Uplift Green Smoothie, 75

Cucumbers
Crunchy Summer Salad, 85
Quinoa and Arugula Salad
with Vegetables, 82
Simple Base Salad, 133

D

Dates
Chocolate Energy Bites, 136
Nutty Blueberry Smoothie, 143

E

Eggplants
Roasted Eggplant Ragù, 119–120

Eggs
Apple-Chia Power Muffins, 69–70
Best Turkey Burgers, 117
Butternut Squash Nest Eggs, 68
Crispy Chicken Tenders, 123–124
Fluffiest Raspberry Pancakes, 72–73
Hearty Black Bean Burgers, 86–87
Lazy Day Italian Wedding Soup, 109
Muffin Tin Frittatas, 76–77
Roasted Vegetable Fried Rice, 96–97
Roasted Vegetable Grain
Bowl, 90–91
Shakshuka, 80
Warm Green Lentil Salad, 118

F

Fish
Baked Mustard Salmon, 116

Fruits. See also specific
Dark Chocolate Dipper, 140

G

Grains. See also specific
Chicken Tikka Masala Grain
Bowl, 94–95
Creamy Masoor Dal Grain
Bowl, 92–93
Crispy Falafel Bowl, 98–99
Roasted Eggplant Ragù, 119–120

Green beans
Crunchy Summer Salad, 85

H

Hemp seeds
Chocolate Energy Bites, 136
Herbs, fresh. *See also specific*
Simple Base Salad, 133

L

Lentils
Creamy Masoor Dal Grain Bowl, 92–93
Crispy Falafel Bowl, 98–99
Lentil-Spinach Fritters, 81
Warm Green Lentil Salad, 118
Lettuce
Shrimp Tacos with Black
Bean Salad, 121–122
Limes
Cilantro-Lime Rice, 128
Roasted Sweet Potato "Hummus," 129
30-Minute Chicken Pho, 112–113

M

Melons
Coconut-Melon Cooler, 141
Mint
Best Turkey Burgers, 117
Coconut-Melon Cooler, 141
Warm Green Lentil Salad, 118
Mushrooms
Roasted Eggplant Ragù, 119–120
Sautéed Mushroom and
Quinoa Bowl, 100

N

Nuts
Apple-Chia Power Muffins, 69–70
Connor's "Cereal" Granola, 71
Creamy Chocolate Oatmeal, 74
Creamy Vanilla Cashew Milk, 148
Crunchy Summer Salad, 85

Quinoa and Arugula Salad
with Vegetables, 82
Roasted Beet Salad with Orange
and Avocado, 132
Simple Base Salad, 133

O

Oats
Chocolate Energy Bites, 136
Connor's "Cereal" Granola, 71
Creamy Chocolate Oatmeal, 74
Onions
Chicken Bone Broth, 106–107
Chicken Tikka Masala Grain Bowl, 94–95
Creamy Masoor Dal Grain Bowl, 92–93
Lentil-Spinach Fritters, 81
Quick Pickled Red Onions, 150
Roasted Vegetable Chili, 110–111
Roasted Vegetable Fried Rice, 96–97
Roasted Vegetable Grain Bowl, 90–91
Shrimp Tacos with Black
Bean Salad, 121–122
Spicy Tomato Salsa, 149
30-Minute Chicken Pho, 112–113
Oranges
Roasted Beet Salad with Orange
and Avocado, 132

P

Parsley
Crispy Falafel Bowl, 98–99
Hearty Black Bean Burgers, 86–87
Roasted Eggplant Ragù, 119–120
Shakshuka, 80
Shrimp Tacos with Black
Bean Salad, 121–122
Pepita seeds
Connor's "Cereal" Granola, 71
Peppers
Crunchy Summer Salad, 85
Hearty Black Bean Burgers, 86–87

V

Vegetables. *See also specific*

Roasted Vegetable Fried
Rice, 96–97

Roasted Vegetable Grain Bowl, 90–91

Y

Yogurt

Chicken Tikka Masala Grain Bowl, 94–95

Z

Zucchini

Best Turkey Burgers, 117

Connor's Chicken Soup, 104–105

One-Pot Chicken and Quinoa, 83–84

Roasted Summer Vegetables, 131

Roasted Vegetable Chili, 110–111

30-Minute Chicken Pho, 112–113

Index

Acknowledgments

I would not be sitting here today writing this book if it wasn't for my husband, Brian, who shows me nothing but love, support, faith, and encouragement in all that I do. Brian, I am truly grateful to call you my husband.

My son, Connor, has been my inspiration for many of the recipes in this book. Connor, you are my greatest joy, inspiration, and motivation. Thank you also to my daughter, who is currently growing in my belly, for putting up with the most exciting and fulfilling yet chaotic time in my life. We can't wait to meet you.

To my amazing sister and brother, who are better cooks than I am, I hope this book makes you proud. I look up to you both like no one else.

Many thanks to my family and friends for all of your love and never-ending support.

From professors to dietitians to all the incredible professionals I have had the honor to learn from and work with, you inspire me to become a better dietitian every day.

Last but not least, I want to take this opportunity to thank each and every client of Chelsea Nutrition who has trusted and supported me from day one. You are what keeps me going.

About the Author

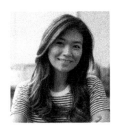 **Jennifer Maeng** holds a Bachelor of Science in Nutrition and Dietetics and a Master of Science in Clinical Nutrition from New York University. She completed her dietetics internship at New York Presbyterian Hospital and went on to specialize in adult clinical nutrition at New York Presbyterian Columbia University Medical Center and NYU Langone Health.

As a clinical dietitian, Jennifer has extensive experience working with a wide range of medical conditions. As a former chef and a restaurateur, Jennifer uses her broad clinical and culinary knowledge to help guide her clients in making lasting lifestyle changes. Her clients range from busy professionals trying to juggle work, life, and health to those who have been recently discharged from the hospital with complicated medical conditions.

When Jennifer is not seeing patients or clients at her private practice, Chelsea Nutrition, she spends her time with her son going to parks and museums. She also loves to go for long runs on the West Side Highway and test new recipes on her husband.